Autologous Stem Cell Transplant
Companion Book

Jonathan I. Angulo

Copyright © 2024, Jonathan I. Angulo

All rights reserved. Without limiting the rights under copyright reserved above, no part of this publication may be reproduced, stored in or introduced into a retrieval system, or transmitted, in any form, or by any means (electronic, mechanical, photocopying, recording, or otherwise) without the prior written permission of the author. This book is licensed for your personal use only. This book may not be re-sold or given away to other people. If you would like to share this book with another person, please purchase an additional copy for each person. The publication/use of any trademarks is not authorized, associated with, or sponsored by the trademark owners. Legal action will be pursued if this is breached.

Cover Art: Jaime Velasco
Cover Design: Graphicsmedium

ISBN: 979-8-9877323-4-2
First Printing, 2024

anguloauthor.com

Autologous Stem Cell Transplant
Companion Book

Jonathan I. Angulo

Disclaimer

This book is meant to be used as a refence only. It is not meant to provide medical advice to anyone. No sponsorship was received from any resources or products mentioned in this book. Normal laboratory values can vary from laboratory to laboratory, and values listed in the glossary should not be considered as 100 percent accurate; please consult the values listed on your own laboratory results for accuracy.

Although there are other medical conditions for which an **autologous stem cell transplant** might be indicated, multiple types of cancer are the main conditions for which it's used. Therefore, this book focuses mostly on advice for patients and caregivers of patients with cancer. However, regardless of your medical condition, the autologous **stem cell transplant** process and care is very similar, and you will find this book useful despite your medical condition.

Caution should be taken not to confuse the main purpose of this book, which is meant to help patients about to undergo an autologous stem cell transplant and not an **allogenic stem cell transplant**. An allogenic stem cell transplant differs a lot, and the advice from this book will not be of much help for patients undergoing that procedure.

Last but not least, it should be noted that different doctors and different facilities have their own way of doing things. The timeline in which procedures might happen might differ due to their own preferences or guidelines. Likewise, different medical conditions might require additional or less testing, procedures, medications, or medical care, before, during and after the transplant.

Acknowledgments

In all humility, I must express that this book owes its existence to my deep passion for the healthcare field and the invaluable experiences I've gained as a healthcare professional. My own battle with cancer, which began in 2022, exposed me to the world of autologous stem cell transplants, inspiring me to pen these pages in the hopes of guiding patients and caregivers through the challenges that lie ahead.

I extend heartfelt gratitude to my editor, Eric Braun, whose unwavering support has been a great pillar in bringing not just this but two other books to life. It's worth mentioning that he donated his own time to help make this book a reality. Similarly, I must expend my gratitude to Jaime Velasco, who donated his own time to create the picture used in the front cover.

Special thanks are also due to Dr. Raghuveer Ranganathan and Dr. John Khoury, who generously devoted their time to ensure the medical accuracy of the content within these pages.

Last but not least, my heartfelt appreciation goes out to my family and my extended ERB work-family, who are always there to support me through the ups and downs. Love you all.

AUTOLOGOUS STEM CELL TRANSPLANT

Learn to use a QR code

1 Open your camera on your device and point it at the QR code.

2 Wait for your device's camera to recognize and scan the QR code.

3 Click the banner/notification/open link when it appears on your device's screen.

4 Information associated with the QR code will automaticall load.

Note: Older devices may require you to download an app to scan the QR code.

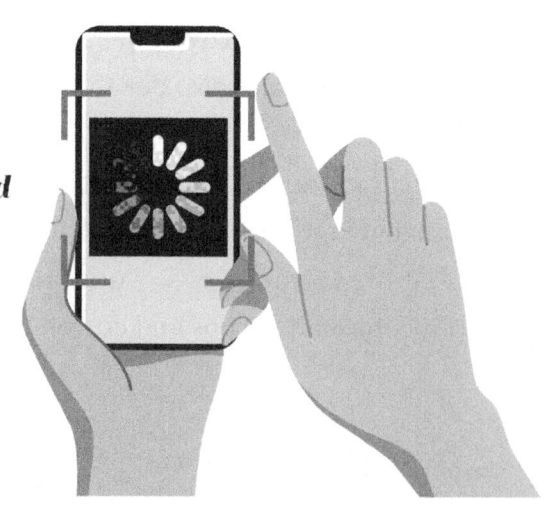

Table of Contents

Introduction	XI
How to Use this Book	XIII
Emergency Information	1
Insight for Caregivers	3
Insight for Patients	17
Useful Items for Men	31
Useful Items for Women	32
Useful Resources	34
Daily Logs	37
Glossary	95
Game Instructions	103
Answer Key	109
Other Books by the Author	116
About the Author	117

Introduction

Whether you are a patient or the caregiver of a patient about to undergo an autologous stem cell transplant, I'm glad you have come across this book.

As a former autologous stem cell transplant recipient, I know how stressful it can be to prepare for this new challenge in our path to get healed. I often hear questions of people asking how to prepare for it. So, I decided to make this book with the hopes that it could help answer those questions and provide other useful information as well.

The purpose of this book is to be of help before, during, and after the transplant. It does not tell my own story—there are plenty of other books out there in which people share theirs. This book is meant to serve as a companion for you to take to the hospital with you and log important information in it.

It is imperative to be on top on your care by logging details such as your daily laboratory values, symptoms, and emotions. By doing that, you'll be able to see how you're improving day by day.

In addition to being a place to log that important information, this book also includes resources that will be useful at the right time. For example, it includes a list of useful items to take with you to the hospital. It includes some insight for both the patient and their caregivers as to what to expect and how to prepare for the upcoming challenges. The are also some **QR codes** that will take you to online resources where you can learn more about different important topics.

A stem cell transplant is a hard treatment to go through. It will bring a lot of challenges and difficult times, and it will test both the patient as well as their caregivers in ways not experienced before. Let's get you on the right path to be a little better prepared for it.

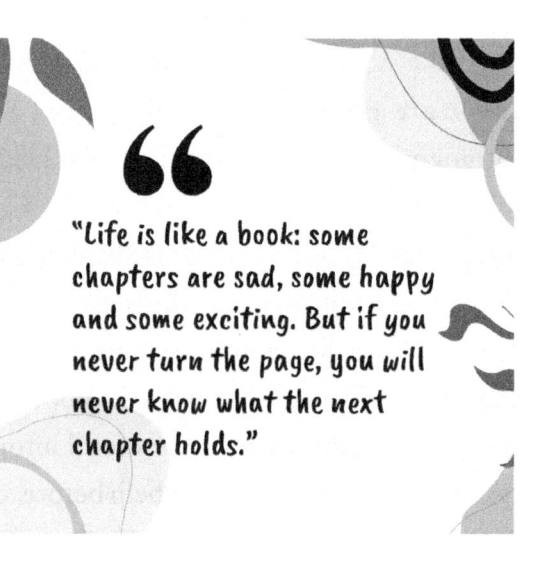

> "Life is like a book: some chapters are sad, some happy and some exciting. But if you never turn the page, you will never know what the next chapter holds."

How to Use this Book

This book is organized in the following way:

We The section after this one is a space to include vital emergency information about the patient. During the hospital stay, the patient's memory and attention span could become less than optimal. This might be due to an expected side effect from some of the medications administered or to simple exhaustion, which means important information such as allergies, current medications, or emergency contact information might not be easy to recall. That is why I encourage you to fill out this section to the best of your ability before the patient gets admitted to the hospital.

Next comes two sections that lay out what to expect before, during, and after the transplant. One is addressed to the caregiver and one to the patient.

Following that you will find two lists of useful items for the patient take to the hospital in order to have a more comfortable stay. Those lists are derived from items that I took to the hospital as well as from feedback gathered from other patients. One list is tailored for men and one for women.

The "Useful Resources" section is next. Here you will find QR codes that will direct you to hand-picked sources that provide useful information for before, during, and after the transplant.

Next is the longest section of the book, the "Daily Logs," where you will log important information on a daily basis. The first page provides an example of how to fill out this section. Pay close attention to that example so you can get the most out of your logs. This section is divided in the following way:

- Vital Signs section: You will most likely have your vital signs taken several times during each day. I have included this section for you to log in those values here both during the morning and in the evening.
- Laboratory Values section: You will also have blood drawn on a daily basis. In this section I have included the most important laboratory values that you should keep an eye on.
- Symptoms Experienced section: Throughout the hospital stay, you will experience variable symptoms. Most of the symptoms you will experience will begin to appear once your blood counts begin to drop. It's important to monitor your symptoms that way you can tell the doctors how you are feeling, and can compare how you feel if they give you medications to help ease those symptoms.
- Games section: It's imperative to distract yourself during the hospital stay. I have included some games that I think will help in keeping you distracted, as well as they will help you keep your mind sharp. The games get progressively more challenging. If you are

unsure of how to play any of the games, there's a "Game Instructions" section at the end of the book. There's also an "Answer Key" section at the end of the book. Have fun!
- Other Notes section: This is free text area for you to write down anything you will like. You might write down how you are feeling emotionally; any questions you might have towards the nurse or the doctor; if you had any blood or **platelets** transfusion; who came to visit you today. Anything you would like.

Finally, you will find the "Glossary." Any words that are **bolded** will appear in the glossary.

EMERGENCY INFORMATION

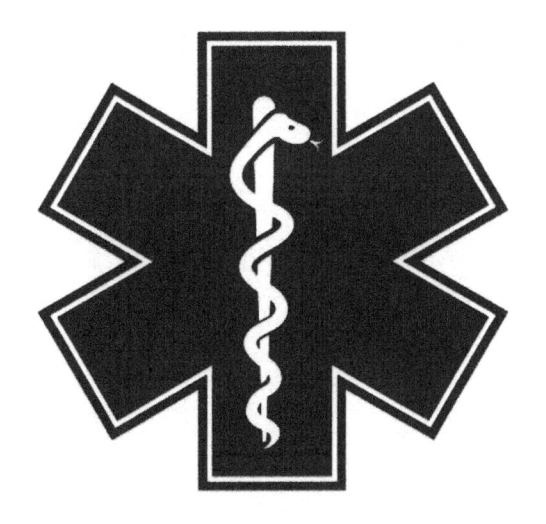

FOLD ME

Autologous Stem Cell Transplant

Name: _____ D.O.B. _____ / _____ / _____

Allergies: _____
_____
_____

Medical History: _____
_____
_____

Surgical History: _____
_____
_____

Medications: _____
_____
_____

Others: _____
_____
_____

Emergency Contacts: _____
_____
_____
_____

Insight for Caregivers

As the caregiver of a cancer patient, you are probably used to seeing the patient go through a lot of ups and downs. You probably know that after having chemotherapy, the patient will experience tiredness, stomach issues, mouth sores, a cloudy mind, sadness, and other symptoms. You also know that it will last for a few days, and then the patient might get to feel better before the next treatment.

Those experiences have prepared you for the new challenges that await before, during, and after the transplant. However, there will of course be new experiences that you will have to prepare yourself for. That way you are well informed and can provide support to the patient.

Before the Transplant

Let's give you a rundown of what you can expect before the transplant.

One of the first things the doctors will need is to ensure the patient is fit to undergo the transplant. For this, the patient will need to have a lot of blood tests, x-rays, and medical clearances often obtained by seeing the heart and lungs specialists.

Once the patient gets cleared to undergo the stem cell transplant journey, the patient will need to prepare to have their stem cells collected.

Now, here's something important to note. While I discuss hospital admissions throughout the book, not all patients undergoing the transplant process will be admitted to the hospital. This could be due to personal preference or the recommendation of their doctor. Some patients opt for outpatient treatment, which means they'll need to visit the hospital or a doctor's office daily. There, they'll have their blood drawn and vital signs checked, they'll receive chemotherapy and other necessary medications, and then they'll head home to rest. While some patients successfully complete the entire process on an outpatient basis, it's crucial to understand that if a patient develops a fever or falls ill at any point, they'll likely need to be admitted to the hospital for the remainder of the treatment.

First, there will be some chemotherapy administered to the patient that is meant to displace their stem cells from the bone marrow inside of the bones and into the veins throughout the body. That way they can be collected in the near future. This chemotherapy is usually a one-time event that lasts for about one hour and is often uneventful. It'll be administered into the veins of the patient via an IV or an existing chemotherapy port.

Second, the patient will need daily injections of a medication to boost the body's production of stem cells. This type of medications, known as Granulocyte Colony Stimulating Factors (G-CSF), work by stimulating the bone marrow to increase stem cell production. These injections are easy to self-administer at home, although sometimes the doctor may prefer the patient to receive them at the office. This process usually lasts 10 or more days. The patient will likely experience bone pain due to these injections, so it's important to prepare for this and ask the doctor for pain medication ahead of time. A common medication given for this type of pain is Loratadine (brand name Claritin). While typically used for seasonal allergies, it can also help alleviate bone marrow pain. Additionally, the patient might be started on medications (such as **antibiotics**) to prevent infections before the collection process begins.

Next, the patient will return to the hospital or be sent to another facility to have a new intravenous line inserted into the large veins of the chest cavity. This line, called an **apheresis line**, is more complex than a chemotherapy port or a regular IV. Initially, it will be used to collect the stem cells into a machine, and afterwards, it will serve to administer drugs throughout the entire hospital stay. An apheresis line is more effective than lines placed in the arms because it allows for easier and safer collection of stem cells from the larger veins, which can accommodate a greater flow of blood and fluids in and out of the body.

The collection process lasts 4 or 5 hours and might need to be completed over the course of more than one day if not enough cells are collected. There a several reasons why a patient might not be able to collect enough cells in one day, so please be ready for this possibility and do not let the patient get discouraged by it. It might be that they recently finished chemotherapy and their bone marrow is a little debilitated by it, it could also be that the patient is an older person and their bone marrow doesn't usually produce a lot of stem cells anymore, or perhaps the patient didn't get the daily injections to boost stem cells production before the collection day. These reasons, as well as many other ones, could play a role, but know that patients do have good outcomes even if they took more than one day to collect the needed cells. If not enough cells are collected the first day, the patient might be given a different type of injection to help their stem cells be collected easier; these injections have a medication similar to the one the patient received as an intravenous infusion before the first collection.

The collection process is uneventful most of the time, but it's just a long process, so bring some books or snacks for the patient. A common side effect during or after the collection process is some numbness or tingling in the hands or feet due to a medication administered during the collection to help preserve the collected cells. Be sure to let the nurses know if the patient experiences this side effect. Once all cells are collected, the hospital will safely store them until the day of the transplant.

Now, before the patient gets admitted to the hospital, the hospital will possibly ask about who will be the caregiver for the patient. The caregiver needs to live within a certain distance of the patient (if they do not live in the same house), and they need to be available at first call to take the patient to the hospital after discharge for follow-ups. It's also a possibility that the patient will feel too weak after discharge, and the caregiver might need to help them with activities of daily living such as walking, bathing, eating, toileting, staying on top of bills, taking medications, and so on. Once the patient's blood counts begin to rise and maintain steadily in a safe range (usually by about day +30), then the patient will begin to feel better and be able to care for themselves.

During the Transplant

Once the patient is admitted to the hospital, the duration of their **conditioning chemotherapy** varies depending on the specific regimen that the doctor has chosen for the patient. It could span as little as one day, though seven or more days is not uncommon. These days of constant chemo are usually called "minus" days, with the day the patient gets their stem cells infused being "Day Zero." All days afterward are called "plus" days.

For example, if a patient will have conditioning chemo for a total of 7 days, then the day the patient gets admitted to the hospital will be called "Day -7," the next day will be "Day -6," and so on until the patients gets their stem cells infused, which will be "Day 0." From then on, all of the following days will have a "+" before them. Day +1, +2, +3, and so on.

An interesting note, stem cell transplant recipients often refer to "Day 0" as their new birthday. Many patients celebrate this "re-birthday" yearly as a day to remember those difficult times and the long way they have come since "Day 0" occurred. But not only patients celebrate it; some hospitals even bring cakes and celebrate it with patients while they are in the hospital receiving their stem cells infusion. Isn't this a nice memorable moment?

The patient will almost certainly have blood drawn the day they are admitted. It's also highly likely that they will receive some chemotherapy that same day. You can expect the patient to be connected to intravenous fluids 24/7, which might make it difficult for the patient to use the restroom, shower, and sleep, so please be supportive of the patient.

As days go by and more chemotherapies are administered, expect the patient to experience side effects such as nausea, vomiting, headaches, loss of appetite, weight gain/loss, fatigue, depression, mouth sores, diarrhea, or other symptoms. The closer the patient gets to finishing all of the chemotherapies that are planned, the more symptoms the patient might begin to experience. I encourage you to share any and all experienced symptoms with the nurses, even if the patient doesn't want to share them. It's important for the doctors to know.

The infusion of the stem cells is almost always a quick and uneventful process. However, there's a very slim possibility of adverse reactions due to the **preservative DMSO** used to store the cells. Just like with any drug, our body might not respond well to it. In the rare case of adverse reactions, the hospital may need to administer medications to the patient to decrease these reactions and ensure the safe administration of the stem cells. Due to that possibility, it's likely that the patient will receive some medications beforehand to reduce the chances of any adverse reactions to the stem cells, such as nausea, vomiting, diarrhea, rashes, itchy skin, fever, shortness of breath, dizziness, or a feeling of tightness in the throat.

Infusing the stem cells will take about 30 minutes, and they are administered like any other drug via the intravenous line. Once the infusion is complete, the patient will probably feel sleepy and may want to nap. A nurse will keep a close watch and monitor the patient for a few hours after the stem cells are infused, taking vital signs multiple times during this period. Here's a fun fact: the infusion of the stem cells has a very distinct smell due to the preservative; some people describe it as resembling garlic, while others liken it to the scent of corn. What will you smell?

Unfortunately, about three days after the patient receives their stem cells, their original **white blood cells**, red blood cells, platelets, and other cells will drop to nearly zero. That's when the worst symptoms begin. The decrease in these cells is due to the chemotherapy received before the stem cells infusion, as it takes this long for the chemotherapy to kill those cells. This decrease in white blood cells causes the immune system to shut down, leading to many of the symptoms experienced.

Blood counts begin to rise again around Day +10 or +11. At this point, the patient may start feeling more like themselves and might be discharged to go home. The hospital will most likely remove any intravenous lines before the patient is discharged.

Before the patient's blood counts begin to rise again, they may need transfusions of red blood cells or platelets. They might also require antibiotics and **antifungal** medications to prevent infections, as their immune system will be almost non-existent. Most infections are caused by the harmless bacteria that live in our gut. Although these bacteria (also known as the **gut microbiome**) usually help us, they might become opportunistic and cause infections. If an infection originates in the gut, the patient might experience symptoms such as severe **abdominal pain**, diarrhea, foul-smelling **feces**, watery diarrhea, chills, fever, and body aches. However, since the immune system also plays a role in the normal structure of our feces, the patient might experience loose stools or diarrhea without necessarily having an infection. That's why it's important to inform the nurses or doctors about any symptoms, so they can closely monitor the patient and check for an infection.

On that same note, while the patient's blood counts are close to zero, they might get injections to boost production of white blood cells, just like the injections given before the collection process. Also, they will probably be directed to clean their entire body with special wipes at least once daily to prevent infections. During this time of low blood counts, the patient might not want to eat, walk, or shower, they might sleep a lot, or develop mouth sores that will make it hard to eat.

Please be patient, supportive, and understanding with the patient during this time. It's normal for some patients to have a lot of accidents due to the diarrhea. Even though it might hurt to see them go through this period, the patient doesn't have a lot of energy and might not be willing to do much other than sleep. It is okay to just sit in silence and be there for them.

There are things that you could do to make the patient and yourself feel better during the stay. For example, some hospitals offer resources for both the patient or the caregiver. Take advantage of them. Some hospitals have a physical therapist come and help the patient with daily exercises, some hospitals offer music therapy, or psychology sessions. Similarly, doing little things like opening the blinds and letting the sunlight come in might also help you and the patient. Try to eat together with the patient, which helps strengthen the bond and boosts the morale of the patient. At nighttime, try to go home and sleep there. The change of scenery might prove very beneficial to you, and you will feel more energized and with a clearer mind to take on the challenges of the next day. It'll be really tiring and uncomfortable for you to sleep at the hospital with all the beeping from machines, lights being on, nurses coming to check the patient at nighttime. Overall, it's a very uncomfortable place to sleep. Please take care of yourself as well, that way you can feel energized and ready to provide good care to the patient the next day.

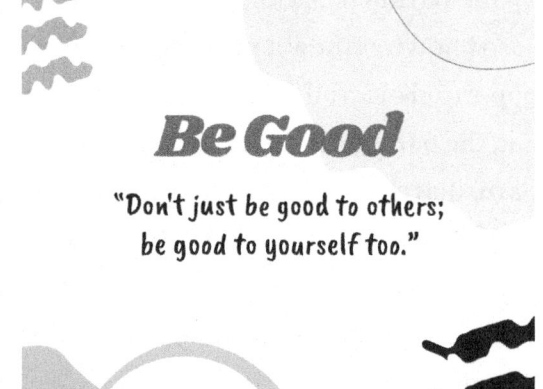

Be Good

"Don't just be good to others; be good to yourself too."

AFTER THE TRANSPLANT

Once this worst ride is over, there will be other challenges to go through. I'm sorry, I wish I could tell you it will all be back to normal right away, but it won't.

The patient will need to have some special care. This includes special food, limited visitors, a clean home, and little or no contact with animals, flowers, or dust, which can carry infections that might be easily picked up by the patient. This is due to the patient having a very weak immune system and needing to take as many precautions as possible to limit any infections. Food that's not cooked properly might be harmful, and some fruits and vegetables that are known to carry certain bacteria will need to be avoided. Also, some foods are not recommended because the patient's gastrointestinal system will not be ready to process them just yet. Some doctors are not so strict about the patient following a careful diet after discharge, but others are very cautious and prefer the patient to wait a longer period of time before "letting his or her guard down" about certain foods. In the end, I recommend you to look at the resources I have included and make your own conclusions and decisions about what's best for the patient's care, and discuss it with the doctor ahead of time.

For example, if the patient is not told to avoid certain foods, eating at restaurants, or ordering take out, ask yourself these questions:

- Do you really believe that restaurants take the highest standards of hygiene while preparing food?
- Do you think that all foods purchased at the grocery store or at the local market are free of harmful bacteria? Or that any and all bacteria can be properly removed by just washing the produce?

I'm pretty sure you answered "no" to at least one those questions—I surely did. Because of this logic, it's recommended that the patient only eats home cooked meals, as one can be sure to properly clean and cook the meals to the proper temperatures to kill harmful bacteria. Similarly, the patient should avoid certain foods or produce that can't be properly cleaned (like strawberries, berries, spinach, lettuce, tree nuts, etc.)

On a similar note, it's also common for the patient to be prescribed several medications to take home in order to prevent infections. These medications may include a mix of **antivirals**, antifungals, and antibiotics. Given their weakened immune system, these additional precautions are necessary. It's not uncommon for patients to be advised to continue taking these medications for several months as a preventive measure. Or some patients might be told to take them only for a few days or months. The duration and number of medications given as a preventive measure varies depending on the doctor's preference and the health status of the patient. For example, older patients or patients with additional health conditions might be put on more medications or be told to take them for a longer period of time. It also depends on how long the patient's defenses (white blood cell counts) take to go up to acceptable levels and continue steadily in those levels.

During this time, the patient will be feeling very fatigued and sleepy. It also becomes harder to think or concentrate on things. This is known as brain fog, and it can last for months for some people. Their sex drive is also affected during this time. Even watching television, walking, sitting, or talking might be tiring. This is the time when it's important for you to be supportive and understanding, and volunteer to help the person to the restroom, change their clothes, help them shower if needed, and feed them. Every patient is different, but it's likely that a patient will need a lot of help until about Day +30 or even later than that.

Once discharged home, the patient might need to be taken to the hospital for consultation and blood work once or twice a week, which can go on for about a month depending on the patient's lab results and their overall improvement. Depending on how well the patient is progressing, their visits to the doctor will begin to be spaced out longer and longer. By Day +30, they might only need to go see the doctor once a week or even less frequently than that. Nevertheless, the patient will be on a close watch until they reach Day +100.

It's very probable that the patient will have another **PET scan** before Day +100. They might also be started on some maintenance chemotherapy before the Day +100 mark. That is usually a low-dose chemo that is given for some patients to increase the chances of the cancer not coming back.

Now, at about six months after the stem cell transplant the patient might be instructed to begin getting some vaccinations again. Due to the high-dose chemotherapy received at the hospital, the patients are considered "never vaccinated" and will need certain **inactivated vaccines** (such as **Tdap, Influenza,** COVID-19, etc.) at specific intervals to gain immunity to diseases. Please consult the oncologist on when the patient should begin getting re-vaccinated and which vaccines they should receive first. Make sure to have this conversation with the oncologist sooner rather than later, to ensure the patient doesn't fall behind schedule. However, there may be exceptions to the usual guidelines, particularly for older patients, who may need to start vaccinations earlier. Some **live vaccines** (such as **MMR, Varicella**, etc.) cannot be received before the 12-month or 24-month marks after the transplant for safety precautions, as in rare cases, they might cause the patient to develop the disease.

On that same note, it's a good idea for caregivers and other people living in the same household as the patient to get vaccinated. Since the patient has no defenses, it's easy to get sick from diseases brought home by others. Particularly if the patient will receive their transplant during the cold and flu season, household members should vaccinate against influenza, COVID-19, and Tdap. A small act, such as getting vaccinated, could go a long way in helping the patient avoid any disease that could hinder their prompt recovery.

As you can see, there will be a lot of challenging times that await you and the patient. It's important that you as the caregiver also take care of yourself, both physically and mentally. It will be a lot to take on some days, and you will feel very powerless and stressed during those times.

One way you can learn how to be more prepared for the upcoming challenges, as well as get some other answers, is by joining a support group for caregivers where you can learn from other caregivers and ask for advice. There are some good ones on Facebook.

Self-care is important. You can't help the patient if you're not feeling well, or if you're not cool as a cucumber. It's okay to say you need a day off and have someone else take care of the patient. It's okay to feel overwhelmed and seek a break. It's okay to seek a counselor or talk with someone about how you are feeling. You will not be a bad wife, husband, mother, daughter, son, friend, etc., for identifying that it might be too much for you some days and taking some time for yourself. So please, pay attention to how you are feeling and what you need. Attend to your needs, that way you can continue taking care of the patient.

Insight for Caregivers

The QR codes below will take you to useful websites that contain information for caregivers. Also see the "Useful Resources" section.

[QR code] Information on the role of the caregiver

[QR code] The importance of caregivers

[QR code] Caregiver resources and support

[QR code] Advice for caregivers

[QR code] Caregivers peer-to-peer support

Facebook Support Groups:

[QR code] Caregivers of Bone Marrow, Stem Cell, & Cord Blood Transplant Survivors

[QR code] Transplant Caregivers – Partners for Life

Insight for Patients

Preparing to undergo a stem cell transplant is not an easy process. It might be that you have never achieved remission and your doctors are recommending this treatment to increase your changes of doing so. Or perhaps you were in remission for a couple of years but unfortunately relapsed, and now this treatment is being suggested to get you in remission again.

Whatever your case might be, I can almost be certain that you're nervous and wondering if this is the right choice to make, as well as if you are ready for the challenges that this procedure will bring to your life.

I cannot tell you if it's the right call for your particular case, but I can share with you some statistics of the success rates of stem cell transplants. Of course, different types of cancer or other diseases have different success rates, and as you have realized by now, every patient is different and every case is unique. However, according to the Cleveland Clinic, a hospital with leading knowledge and investigations about multiple diseases, the most recent data shows that people who undergo a stem cell transplant have a three-year survival rate in the following percentages:

- Hodgkin's lymphoma: About 92 percent of people
- Non-Hodgkin's lymphoma: About 72 percent of people.
- Multiple myeloma: About 79 percent of people.

Stem cell transplants have been in use since 1958, and as you can imagine, they have come a long way since then. Doctors have learned a lot over the years and have developed better ways to ensure the safety of the patients undergoing the procedure. According to the Cleveland Clinic, about 18,000 people in the United States learn each year that they have a disease that a stem cell transplant could cure. In 2020 alone, there were 22,000 stem cell transplants performed worldwide. Diseases such as Multiple Myeloma, Lymphomas, Testicular Cancer, Multiple Sclerosis, and Amyloidosis, are among those diseases for which autologous stem cell transplants might be an option.

Before the Transplant

Now that we have taken care of the statistics, and hopefully gave you a little bit of peace of mind, let's focus on giving you an idea of what to expect before the transplant. I won't get into much detail here because I've already done so in the "Insight for Caregivers" section, which I recommend you read.

In a nutshell, you will probably have to begin getting ready for the transplant the month before you're supposed to be admitted to the hospital. You will need to select someone to be your designated caregiver after you get discharged, you will need to get a bunch of tests done, receive some chemotherapy, get some daily injections to boost your white blood cells counts, get a central or peripheral line (even if you already have a port), and then have your stem cells collected.

During that same month, you are likely to have to go see your primary doctor, a **cardiologist**, and a **pulmonologist** to get medical clearances from them before you have your transplant. They will need to perform some tests to ensure you are okay for that procedure. You will also need to have a bunch of blood drawn for a variety of tests, including one to determine your blood type and others to check for a variety of infectious diseases.

Now, here's an important issue to deal with before your transplant: fertility preservation. It's a possibility that the high dosage chemotherapy that you will receive before the transplant could leave you infertile or unable to have babies. If having a baby is something still in your plans for the future, please talk to your doctor ahead of time. Even children can undergo fertility preservation, so please have this conversation early with your doctors. Fertility preservation could be expensive, but there are companies that offer huge discounts for patients with cancer, so please ask your doctor or the hospital team for their available resources.

On that same note, if you're a female who still gets her period, I suggest you have a conversation with your doctor about if you should take any hormones to stop your period from coming while you undergo the transplant. There are patients who get an injection to help with that; a common one is a called **Lupron**. The reason is that there will be a time when your platelets will be too low and having your period at that time might not be a great idea, as your body is not capable of controlling the bleeding.

Another important piece of advice is to get any legal paperwork taken care of. Now this might be kind of an elephant-in-the-room conversation, but it needs to be had. If you're an adult and you have bills to take care of, or have children who might need to be taken to the doctor or to school, then it's important that you prepare for the worst and hope for the best. What do I mean by that? Well, it's almost certainly that during and after the transplant, you will be feeling highly fatigued or foggy-headed, and your mind will not be at its best for making decisions. That's why it's important that you leave some things in writing ahead of time.

This might mean that you leave some signed letters authorizing a trustable person to pay your bills, or to take your children to school or the doctor. Perhaps you will need to leave your passwords and log-in information for your bank or other websites that you often log into, like for credit cards and utilities. It might also mean that you get prepared for the worst and take care of your living will or advance directive at this point. Again, I know these are sensitive topics, but it's best to think a step ahead and get those things taken care of.

Lastly, one more piece of advice to help you before the transplant: join a support group. You will probably have way more questions than the ones I'm answering in this book. Or you might want to hear about first-hand experiences from other people with your same condition who have undergone a stem cell transplant. Whatever the case might be, it's important to stay connected to others who have already navigated the journey you're about to embark on, because they can provide insight and advice. So, I recommend that you join a Facebook group of people with your condition. I have researched some good ones, and I have included the information for those groups at the end of this section. Please utilize it.

During the Transplant

I want to remind you again to read the "Insight for Caregivers" section, where you can get a good overview of what the hospital stay will be like.

With that being said, let me tell you, this hospital stay is not going to be a joke. It will challenge you and test your strength and patience in ways you have not been tested before. I wish I could sugarcoat it and tell you that it's going to be a breeze, but it's not, and I'm sorry.

If you like going to bed and sleeping in without disruptions, you better start preparing yourself for the opposite. It's not uncommon to be connected to the IV machine and have infusions running all day long, you will probably be awoken once or twice each night by the staff to take your vital signs or give you medications, or by the IV pump machine that randomly begins beeping, "beep, beep, beep" on and on and on. I recommend you bring a blindfold and ear plugs to help you rest as much as possible during the night.

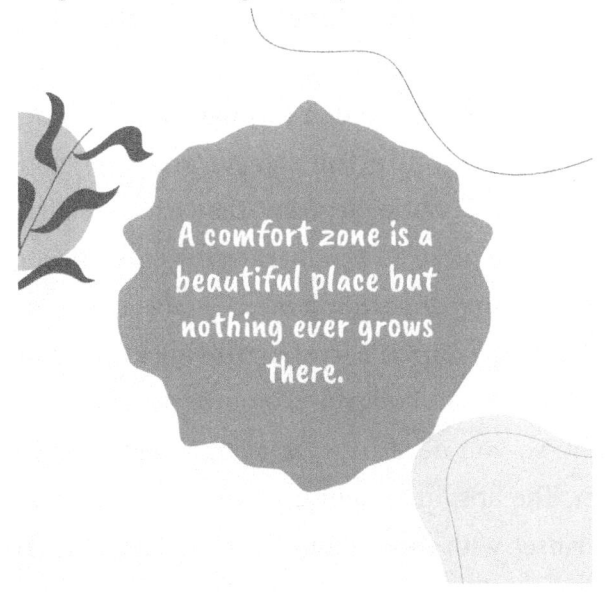

> A comfort zone is a beautiful place but nothing ever grows there.

If you like having a pleasant shower, give up on that idea, too. Because you will have either the central (in your chest) or peripheral (in your arms) intravenous line, and you have to be extra cautious when showering to not get it wet. That means you have to limit your shower time and use a lot of tape and plastic protectors (hopefully provided by the hospital) to cover up the intravenous line during your shower. Now, if you're like me and enjoy a nice, long shower, you will probably lose interest in that after one or two hospital showers and will not even want to shower every day, much less spend a long time doing it. Sadly, it's important that you shower daily because your defenses will be almost non-existent during your stay, and keeping clean through showers helps decrease the odds of any bacteria growing around your body or entering your bloodstream via the intravenous line or any open wounds.

The hospital might provide you with some cleaning wipes to use on your entire body on a daily basis as well. Please use them; they will also decrease the chances of any bacteria becoming opportunistic and getting you sick. The last thing you want is to get sick because of something you could have avoided through simple hygiene. If you're too tired, the nurses can help you shower and wipe your body. You might feel embarrassed, but believe me, they have seen it all.

On that same note, it's imperative to practice good mouth hygiene. This will help reduce the chances of developing mouth sores as well as decrease the chance of bacteria growing inside your mouth. It's very common for patients to develop mouth sores when going through this transplant, so you need to try and be a step ahead of the game to avoid them. The hospital might give you some special medications to do mouth rinses with throughout the day; use them. Also, there's a good mouth rinse called biotène dry mouth oral rinse that helps your mouth stay moisturized. My hospital provided this for me, and I guess it helped because I didn't develop mouth sores. If your hospital doesn't provide it, you can get it at any drug store or online. There's also a natural supplement called Glutasolve (Glutamine) that the nutritionist recommended during my stay; it's a powder taken two times a day that gets dissolved in apple sauce, and it helps reduce the chance of getting mouth sores. I'd recommend you look into it and ask your doctor if you can get it during your stay.

On a similar note: if one of your planned chemo drugs is Evomela (Melphalan), that's the one that's known to cause the mouth sores as well as diarrhea. Doctors usually recommend eating ice chips or sucking on lollipops while getting this chemotherapy infusion in order to help reduce the chances of getting mouth sores.

Diarrhea is also very common, with some patients experiencing really watery diarrhea for days and others just get loose stools for a few days. Depending on your symptoms, the doctor might ask for a stool sample to determine if you have an infection in your digestive system before they can prescribe you with strong medications to stop the diarrhea. It's a common saying among stem cell transplant recipients to tell others during this time to "never trust a fart." That's because diarrhea can cause a lot of accidents, so please be ready for it. A lot of patients purchase their own pampers to take to the hospital with them and wear them daily once diarrhea begins, especially because store-bought ones are usually more comfortable than the ones the hospital might provide you with. My nutritionist at the hospital also recommended Banatrol, a powder that helps with diarrhea, and I recommend you discuss this with your doctor before the hospital stay to see if it'd be a good idea for you to take.

On a final note, while at the hospital you will play an important role in how well and how quickly you recover. It's normal to feel disconnected from the world and lacking in motivation to do things. However, if you let these feelings overtake you, then everything is going to feel more depressing and you will not be helping your recovery. Instead, try to do things that might make you feel better or that might be beneficial for your body. For example, try to wake up and watch the news—that way you feel a little more connected with the outside world. Or make some phone calls or send texts messages. Also, it's highly recommended that you walk during your stay at the hospital. Yes, it might be cumbersome to have to walk while being connected to the IV machine, but still, it will do your body good to get your blood circulating better through your body.

As I've mentioned in previous sections, most of your symptoms will begin around Day +3 (three days after your stem cells are infused). During this time, your appetite will decrease so much that you will find yourself not eating much. I remember I would be so hungry and wanting to eat,

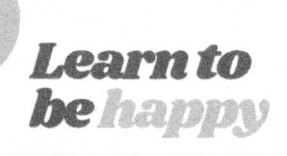

Learn to be happy

Don't wait for things to get easier, simpler, better. Life will always be complicated. Learn to be happy right now. Otherwise you will run out of time.

but when I had the food in front of me, it would take me forever to finish it—I just wasn't feeling it. It's very possible that the taste of some foods might change at this point, so that's another reason why eating becomes less appealing. The thing is, even though you're not hungry, you still need to eat to meet your body demands. I suggest you ask the nurses if they have protein shakes such as Ensure or Orgain for you to drink instead of eating. Orgain was recommended to me because it's friendlier with the gastrointestinal system and is less prone to cause diarrhea. Also, I was told to try to avoid foods that are greasy or spicy, contain lactose, or have a lot of aroma to them. I ate a lot of peanut butter and jelly sandwiches, and that felt better for me.

It's important that you communicate with your doctors or nurses once you begin developing symptoms because they might need to do further testing to ensure you're okay. If you have pain when urinating, or a lot of abdominal pain, blood in your stools or in the toilet paper, diarrhea, dizziness when standing up, headaches, or other symptoms, you should let them know so they can get **blood cultures**, **stool cultures**, or perhaps blood or platelets transfusion. There's no way for them to help you if you do not communicate with them, so please do so even if it's an embarrassing issue. You don't want them to find out about an infection later on when it is more advanced or when your blood counts are way too low. This might make the doctors have to play catch-up to try to help you, and it might also prolong your hospital stay due to complications.

At the end of this long ride, you will get discharged to go home, usually around Day +10 or later. The timing will depend on when your **Neutrophils** (a type of white blood cells) counts have come up to acceptable levels, if other important laboratory results are within acceptable ranges, if you're able to eat, and if you look good overall. As you can imagine, getting discharged will make you feel very happy, but sadly there are other challenges that await you at home, and for quite a few weeks after being discharged.

After the Transplant

Let's explore what life will be like after the hospital.

First of all, I don't think I can express with words how nice and exciting it feels to be able to go home after your hospital stay, which will be about three weeks long in the best-case scenario. Being able to sleep in your bed, watch TV in your room, and shower without any plastic coverings or tape on your body will remind you just how nice all those little things are that we take for granted. Sleeping without any intravenous lines or being awakened by nurses or a machine beeping is just such a nice feeling.

Unfortunately, not everything will be like it was before the transplant. As I mentioned in the "Insight for Caregivers" section, there will be a few things that you will need to be careful about for a few days. You will need constant visits to the doctor for blood work and possibly more blood or platelet transfusions because your doctor will keep you on a close watch until Day +100. However, you will be allowed more freedom way before that as your energy, lab results, appetite, and other markers continue to improve, and you might only need to go to appointments about once a month.

Again, it's important to follow the doctors' instructions very carefully. They might recommend avoiding certain foods at first because they might be too much for your gastrointestinal system to handle soon after the transplant. Do not make the mistake I made and order a pizza a few days after you get home, because you will pay for it with lots of abdominal cramps and diarrhea. Your body is just not ready for those foods yet. Your bowels have shrunk and shriveled, and your gut's ability to process heavy foods has gone down dramatically. You must be kind to your gut after the transplant and have to teach it how to "walk" before it can "run" again. A good way to do this is to begin eating easy-to-digest foods. A common diet to help with this is known as the BRAT diet, which stands for Bread, Rice, Apple sauce, and Toast.

Similarly, you will be asked to refrain from doing activities like going for very long recreational walks, gardening, cleaning your house (yes, you read that right, you will be excused from house chores), having many visitors, and ordering take-out foods, and you will even need to be very careful about how your foods are cooked. All of these restrictions are due to your immune system being almost non-existent when you first get home, so you need to be careful to avoid activities that might take advantage of this temporary weakness and make you sick.

On the same note, you will also be told to exercise—I'm sorry, but you cannot just be a couch potato. You might not be ready for long walks at the park just yet, but you can still do a few laps around your block while wearing a mask. Walking will help you in many ways. It helps give your muscles and bones strength, relieves stress, gives you energy, gives you a change of scenery, encourages your body to work more effectively by circulating your blood more efficiently (which in turn helps you avoid blood clots from developing in your legs, especially if you're an older adult), and gets your lungs to expand more than if you're just lying in bed.

If you follow all of the doctor's advice and are proactive in trying to recover from this hard challenge, you will likely begin feeling like yourself by around Day +30. You might notice an increase of energy, more clearness in your mind, and an overall feeling of being back in your body, if that makes sense. By around Day +40, your digestive system might feel better, more ready to take on heavier meals, and you might be given the green light by your doctor to order take-out or eat other meals like pizza, cheese, or processed meats and breads.

As far as appearance goes, it's very probable that you lost a lot of your hair while at the hospital. Different people will experience different degrees of hair loss, and the types of chemotherapy that you received also plays a factor in how much hair you lose. But in general, you can anticipate significant hair regrowth around the five-month mark after the transplant.

For female patients, you should know that it's likely your period will not come back right away after the transplant. Some patients will get it back between six months to a year after the transplant. On the other hand, some patients will not get it back again and will be pushed into **menopause**. This is most probable if you have your transplant while in your 30s or 40s. It's recommended to follow up with your **gynecologist** if you see that your period is taking long to come back; that way you can get tests done to see if you're in menopause or not.

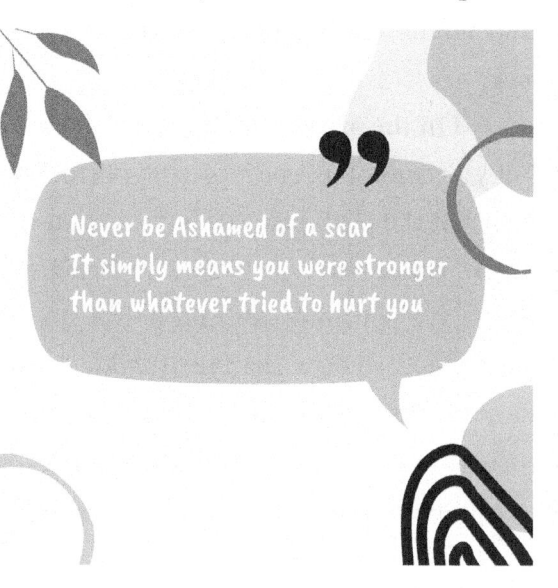

> Never be Ashamed of a scar
> It simply means you were stronger
> than whatever tried to hurt you

As you get closer to Day +100, you might undergo a PET scan to evaluate how you are doing, and you might be started on maintenance chemotherapy. Usually, no sooner than six months after your transplant, you will be instructed to begin getting some vaccinations. Please consult with your doctor about which ones you should get.

One last piece of important advice: please be aware that this process will carry a toll for you as well as for your loved ones around you. It'll be hard for those around you to understand completely how you feel, just as it will be hard for you to understand how difficult it is for your loved ones to see you tired, frustrated, or just not like yourself. Please take the time to talk to a therapist if needed to help you navigate these challenges. You may also want to encourage your loved ones to speak to one if you see them having a hard time enduring the challenges. Help each other out.

Next are some QR codes that will take you to useful websites that contain information for the patient. Also see the "Useful Resources" section.

Facebook Support Groups:

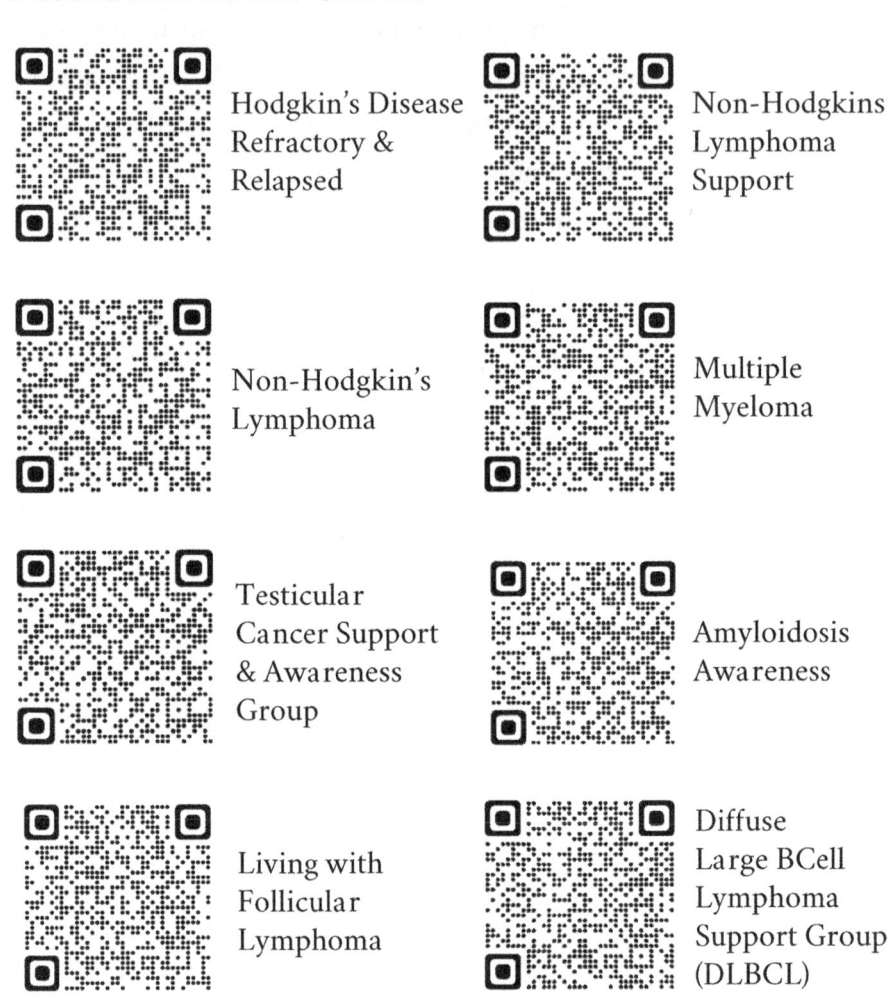

[QR code] Hodgkin's Disease Refractory & Relapsed

[QR code] Non-Hodgkins Lymphoma Support

[QR code] Non-Hodgkin's Lymphoma

[QR code] Multiple Myeloma

[QR code] Testicular Cancer Support & Awareness Group

[QR code] Amyloidosis Awareness

[QR code] Living with Follicular Lymphoma

[QR code] Diffuse Large BCell Lymphoma Support Group (DLBCL)

[QR code] Mantle Cell Lymphoma Support

Useful Items for Men ♂

Leisure	
Books	Laptop/DVDs
iPad	Earphones or headphones
Magazine	Amazon Fire TV stick or similar
Puzzles	Drawing/coloring book

Comfort	
Pillow	Extra underwear (accidents)
Slippers	Hat/beanies (hair loss)
Pajamas and blanket	Lap/folding desk
Family pictures	Eye mask and ear plugs

Toiletries
Rectal cream (will help if you have diarrhea)
Baby wipes (will help if you have diarrhea)
Shampoo and body wash
Disinfecting wipes
Soft toothbrush and toothpaste
Razor and Cologne
Diapers (will help if you have diarrhea)
Central/PICC Line covers with adhesive (can be found at Amazon, useful to be able to shower)

Others
Journal and Snacks
Electronic and Power cord chargers
Dumbbells
Kids' pictures or drawings
Reading glasses (if needed)
Wireless mouse and keyboard
Ensure or *Orgain* nutritional shakes (will help once appetite is lost)
Important medical records (recent scan reports, lab results, name of your doctors, anything else you consider important)

Useful Items for Women ♀

Leisure	
Books	Laptop/DVDs
iPad	Earphones or headphones
Magazine	Amazon Fire TV stick or similar
Puzzles	Drawing/coloring book

Comfort	
Pillow, Slippers, Fan	Extra underwear (accidents)
Baggy shirts/hoodies	Hat/beanies/wigs (hair loss)
Pajamas and blanket	Lap/folding desk
Family pictures	Eye mask and ear plugs

Toiletries
Rectal cream (will help if you have diarrhea)
Baby wipes (will help if you have diarrhea)
Shampoo and body wash
Soft bathroom towel
Soft toothbrush and toothpaste
Razor and Perfume
Central/PICC Line covers with adhesive (can be found at Amazon, useful to be able to shower)

Toiletries continued...
Moisturizing body cream
Makeup and Lip bam
Makeup removal items
Fragrance for room and/or bathroom
Toilet paper
Menstrual hygiene products
Diapers (will help if you have diarrhea)

OTHERS
Journal
Electronic and Power cord chargers
Snacks
Kids' pictures or drawings
Reading glasses (if needed)
Wireless mouse and keyboard
Ensure or *Orgain* nutritional shakes (will help once appetite is lost)
Important medical records (recent scan reports, lab results, name of your doctors, anything else you consider important)

USEFUL RESOURCES

Learn the basis of a stem cell transplant
nmdp.org

Stem cell transplant information
clevelandclinic.org

Information on diseases for which a transplant may be a treatment option
nmdp.org

Another resource with stem cell transplant information
Leukemia & Lymphoma Society

Useful Resources

Information on care after the transplant
nmdp.org

Information on getting re-vaccinated after the transplant
nmdp.org

Information on food safety after the transplant
BeTheMatch.org

Babies After Cancer
Facebook group for females about fertility support after transplant

Conditioning chemotherapy drugs information
Learn about the drugs that will be administered to you
Chemocare.com/druginfo

Daily Logs

Daily Logs

Day: -7　　　　Date: January 9, 2023

VITAL SIGNS

A.M.

Weight: __200__ (lbs.)/ kg.
Blood Pressure: __120/80__
Heart Rate: __80__ bpm
Oxygen Sat: __98__ %
Temperature: __98.6__ (F)/ C

P.M.

Weight: __202__ (lbs.)/ kg.
Blood Pressure: __124/84__
Heart Rate: __88__ bpm
Oxygen Sat: __98__ %
Temperature: __98.6__ (F)/ C

LABORATORY VALUES

WBC: __3.82__
Neutrophils: __2.33__
Hemoglobin: __14.5__
Platelets: __16.5__
Potassium: __3.9__
Calcium: __8.9__
Magnesium: __2.4__
Creatinine: __0.80__
Glucose: __100__
ALT: __24__
AST: __26__
Other ( ): _____

SYMPTOMS EXPERIENCED

Nausea	Y/N	Abdominal Pain	Y/N
Vomiting	Y/N	Shortness of Breath	Y/N
Dizziness	Y/N	Chest Pain	Y/N
Diarrhea	Y/N	Heart Palpitations	Y/N
Loose Stools	Y/N	Headache	Y/N
Mouth Sores	Y/N	Acid Reflux/Heartburn	Y/N
Tired/Fatigued	Y/N	Rash	Y/N

Daily Logs

2	1	4	3
4	3	2	1
1	4	3	2
3	2	1	4

Other Notes:

Today I got admitted. I like my room.

Received chemotherapy today. Felt good except some nausea.

Nurse gave me Ondansetron intravenously and it took away the nausea completely.

Daily Logs

Day: _____   Date: _____

VITAL SIGNS

A.M.
Weight: _____ lbs. / kg.
Blood Pressure: _____
Heart Rate: _____ bpm
Oxygen Sat: _____ %
Temperature: _____ F / C

P.M.
Weight: _____ lbs. / kg.
Blood Pressure: _____
Heart Rate: _____ bpm
Oxygen Sat: _____ %
Temperature: _____ F / C

LABORATORY VALUES

WBC: _____
Neutrophils: _____
Hemoglobin: _____
Platelets: _____
Potassium: _____
Calcium: _____
Magnesium: _____
Creatinine: _____
Glucose: _____
ALT: _____
AST: _____
Other ( ): _____

SYMPTOMS EXPERIENCED

Nausea	Y/N	Abdominal Pain	Y/N
Vomiting	Y/N	Shortness of Breath	Y/N
Dizziness	Y/N	Chest Pain	Y/N
Diarrhea	Y/N	Heart Palpitations	Y/N
Loose Stools	Y/N	Headache	Y/N
Mouth Sores	Y/N	Acid Reflux/Heartburn	Y/N
Tired/Fatigued	Y/N	Rash	Y/N

Daily Logs

4	3	1	
3	4		1
1	2	4	

Other Notes:

Daily Logs

Day: _____ Date: _____

VITAL SIGNS

A.M.

Weight: _____ lbs. / kg.
Blood Pressure: _____
Heart Rate: _____ bpm
Oxygen Sat: _____ %
Temperature: _____ F / C

P.M.

Weight: _____ lbs. / kg.
Blood Pressure: _____
Heart Rate: _____ bpm
Oxygen Sat: _____ %
Temperature: _____ F / C

LABORATORY VALUES

WBC: _____
Neutrophils: _____
Hemoglobin: _____
Platelets: _____
Potassium: _____
Calcium: _____
Magnesium: _____
Creatinine: _____
Glucose: _____
ALT: _____
AST: _____
Other ( ): _____

SYMPTOMS EXPERIENCED

Nausea	Y/N	Abdominal Pain	Y/N
Vomiting	Y/N	Shortness of Breath	Y/N
Dizziness	Y/N	Chest Pain	Y/N
Diarrhea	Y/N	Heart Palpitations	Y/N
Loose Stools	Y/N	Headache	Y/N
Mouth Sores	Y/N	Acid Reflux/Heartburn	Y/N
Tired/Fatigued	Y/N	Rash	Y/N

Daily Logs

B	F	U	A	X	L	O	F	I	G
G	E	A	S	T	R	N	T	I	B
Z	I	W	E	S	T	D	U	X	S
E	Y	C	N	D	H	M	E	O	N
W	B	V	W	D	B	A	U	O	T
I	A	H	H	G	L	T	R	K	R
M	H	L	R	I	H	T	Q	T	S
I	Z	K	I	D	H	B	I	B	T
D	N	W	R	H	R	W	V	V	D
C	M	C	J	N	T	N	E	F	F

EAST   WEST   NORTH   SOUTH

Other Notes:
_____
_____
_____
_____
_____
_____

Daily Logs

Day: _____   Date: _____

VITAL SIGNS

A.M.
Weight: _____ lbs. / kg.
Blood Pressure: _____
Heart Rate: _____ bpm
Oxygen Sat: _____ %
Temperature: _____ F / C

P.M.
Weight: _____ lbs. / kg.
Blood Pressure: _____
Heart Rate: _____ bpm
Oxygen Sat: _____ %
Temperature: _____ F / C

LABORATORY VALUES

WBC: _____
Neutrophils: _____
Hemoglobin: _____
Platelets: _____
Potassium: _____
Calcium: _____
Magnesium: _____
Creatinine: _____
Glucose: _____
ALT: _____
AST: _____
Other ( ): _____

SYMPTOMS EXPERIENCED

Nausea	Y/N	Abdominal Pain	Y/N
Vomiting	Y/N	Shortness of Breath	Y/N
Dizziness	Y/N	Chest Pain	Y/N
Diarrhea	Y/N	Heart Palpitations	Y/N
Loose Stools	Y/N	Headache	Y/N
Mouth Sores	Y/N	Acid Reflux/Heartburn	Y/N
Tired/Fatigued	Y/N	Rash	Y/N

U.S. LICENSE PLATES

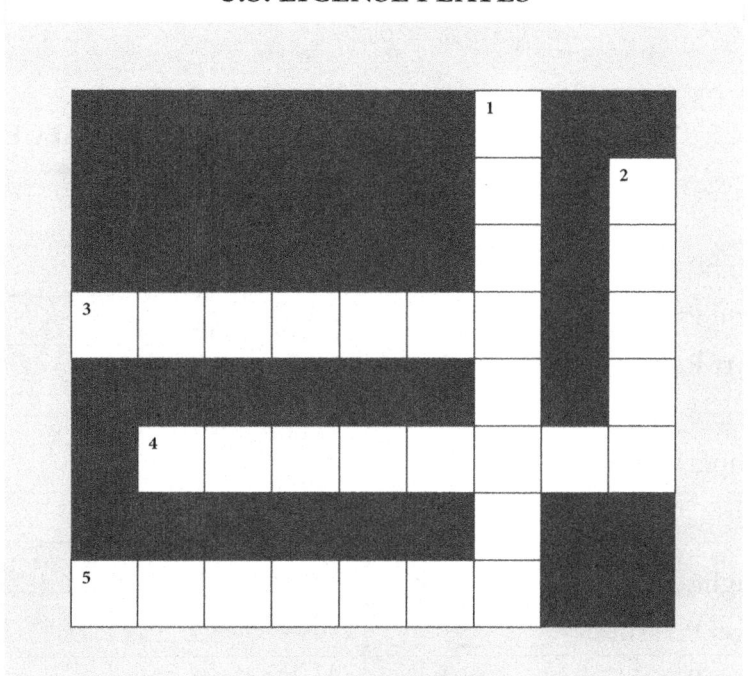

ACROSS:

3. U.S. state that features an orange on its license plate

4. U.S. state that features Abraham Lincoln on its license plate

5. U.S. state that features a peach on its license plate

DOWN:

1. U.S. state that features an archer on its license plate

2. U.S. state that features a lonely star on its license plate

Other Notes:

Daily Logs

Day: _____   Date: _____

VITAL SIGNS

A.M.

Weight: _____ lbs. / kg.
Blood Pressure: _____
Heart Rate: _____ bpm
Oxygen Sat: _____ %
Temperature: _____ F / C

P.M.

Weight: _____ lbs. / kg.
Blood Pressure: _____
Heart Rate: _____ bpm
Oxygen Sat: _____ %
Temperature: _____ F / C

LABORATORY VALUES

WBC: _____
Neutrophils: _____
Hemoglobin: _____
Platelets: _____
Potassium: _____
Calcium: _____
Magnesium: _____
Creatinine: _____
Glucose: _____
ALT: _____
AST: _____
Other ( ): _____

SYMPTOMS EXPERIENCED

Nausea	Y/N	Abdominal Pain	Y/N
Vomiting	Y/N	Shortness of Breath	Y/N
Dizziness	Y/N	Chest Pain	Y/N
Diarrhea	Y/N	Heart Palpitations	Y/N
Loose Stools	Y/N	Headache	Y/N
Mouth Sores	Y/N	Acid Reflux/Heartburn	Y/N
Tired/Fatigued	Y/N	Rash	Y/N

TIC-TAC-TOE

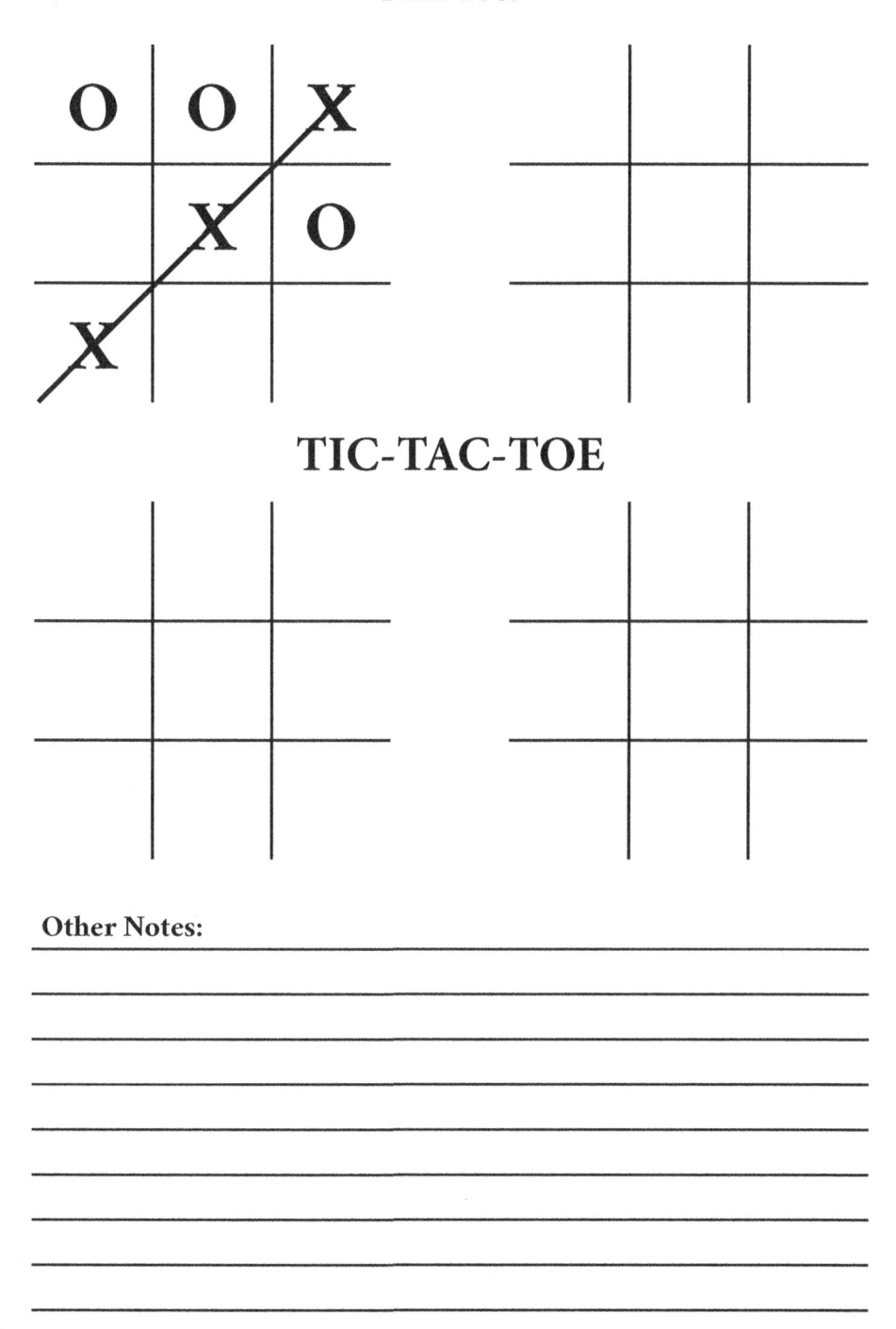

Other Notes:

Daily Logs

Day: _____ Date: _____

VITAL SIGNS

A.M.

Weight: _____ lbs. / kg.
Blood Pressure: _____
Heart Rate: _____ bpm
Oxygen Sat: _____ %
Temperature: _____ F / C

P.M.

Weight: _____ lbs. / kg.
Blood Pressure: _____
Heart Rate: _____ bpm
Oxygen Sat: _____ %
Temperature: _____ F / C

LABORATORY VALUES

WBC: _____
Neutrophils: _____
Hemoglobin: _____
Platelets: _____
Potassium: _____
Calcium: _____
Magnesium: _____
Creatinine: _____
Glucose: _____
ALT: _____
AST: _____
Other (   ): _____

SYMPTOMS EXPERIENCED

Nausea	Y/N	Abdominal Pain	Y/N
Vomiting	Y/N	Shortness of Breath	Y/N
Dizziness	Y/N	Chest Pain	Y/N
Diarrhea	Y/N	Heart Palpitations	Y/N
Loose Stools	Y/N	Headache	Y/N
Mouth Sores	Y/N	Acid Reflux/Heartburn	Y/N
Tired/Fatigued	Y/N	Rash	Y/N

Daily Logs

	4	2	3
2	3	1	4
4			

Other Notes:
_____
_____
_____
_____
_____
_____
_____
_____

Daily Logs

Day: _____   Date: _____

VITAL SIGNS

A.M.

Weight: _____ lbs. / kg.
Blood Pressure: _____
Heart Rate: _____ bpm
Oxygen Sat: _____ %
Temperature: _____ F / C

P.M.

Weight: _____ lbs. / kg.
Blood Pressure: _____
Heart Rate: _____ bpm
Oxygen Sat: _____ %
Temperature: _____ F / C

LABORATORY VALUES

WBC: _____
Neutrophils: _____
Hemoglobin: _____
Platelets: _____
Potassium: _____
Calcium: _____
Magnesium: _____
Creatinine: _____
Glucose: _____
ALT: _____
AST: _____
Other ( ): _____

SYMPTOMS EXPERIENCED

Nausea	Y/N	Abdominal Pain	Y/N
Vomiting	Y/N	Shortness of Breath	Y/N
Dizziness	Y/N	Chest Pain	Y/N
Diarrhea	Y/N	Heart Palpitations	Y/N
Loose Stools	Y/N	Headache	Y/N
Mouth Sores	Y/N	Acid Reflux/Heartburn	Y/N
Tired/Fatigued	Y/N	Rash	Y/N

Daily Logs

C	F	A	T	Q	A	N	O	A	S	C	X
E	Y	F	A	I	T	H	M	X	O	M	Q
S	N	G	X	N	T	R	M	N	Y	R	H
T	C	D	B	G	N	H	T	F	E	W	D
R	D	T	U	X	I	R	M	H	K	C	Z
E	H	P	G	R	O	I	T	O	O	A	Y
N	T	X	Z	L	A	E	V	U	H	E	N
G	K	P	B	S	G	N	R	C	O	X	Y
T	W	T	A	O	W	A	C	T	P	M	R
H	F	U	T	A	G	E	W	E	E	B	G
A	U	W	F	E	G	H	Y	M	R	F	M
L	R	E	S	I	L	I	E	N	C	E	T

| COURAGE | ENDURANCE | FAITH | RESILIENCE |
| HOPE | STRENGTH | CONTROL | TOGETHER |

Other Notes:

_____
_____
_____
_____

Daily Logs

Day: _____   Date: _____

VITAL SIGNS

A.M.

Weight: _____ lbs. / kg.
Blood Pressure: _____
Heart Rate: _____ bpm
Oxygen Sat: _____ %
Temperature: _____ F / C

P.M.

Weight: _____ lbs. / kg.
Blood Pressure: _____
Heart Rate: _____ bpm
Oxygen Sat: _____ %
Temperature: _____ F / C

LABORATORY VALUES

WBC: _____
Neutrophils: _____
Hemoglobin: _____
Platelets: _____
Potassium: _____
Calcium: _____
Magnesium: _____
Creatinine: _____
Glucose: _____
ALT: _____
AST: _____
Other ( ): _____

SYMPTOMS EXPERIENCED

Nausea	Y/N	Abdominal Pain	Y/N
Vomiting	Y/N	Shortness of Breath	Y/N
Dizziness	Y/N	Chest Pain	Y/N
Diarrhea	Y/N	Heart Palpitations	Y/N
Loose Stools	Y/N	Headache	Y/N
Mouth Sores	Y/N	Acid Reflux/Heartburn	Y/N
Tired/Fatigued	Y/N	Rash	Y/N

BODY ORGANS

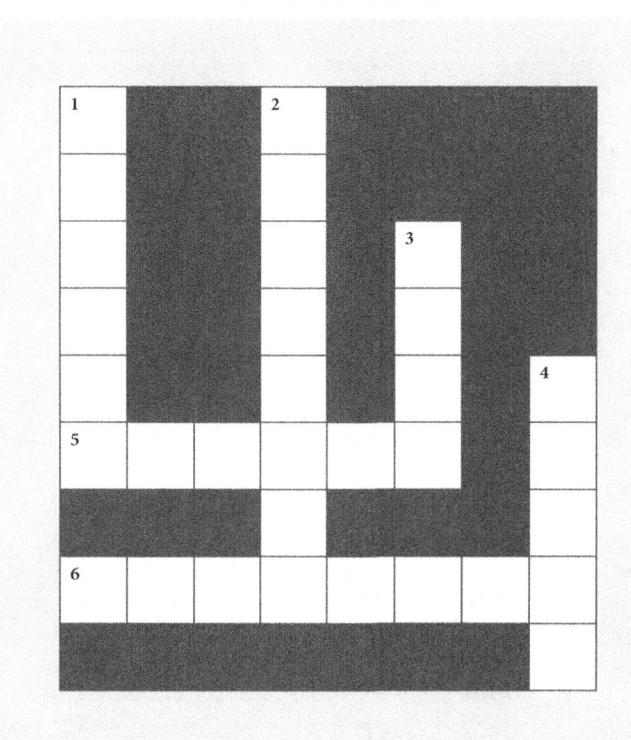

ACROSS:

5. Body organ that helps store and replace red blood cells and immune cells

6. Body organ that is only present in Males

DOWN:

1. Body organ that plays an important role in immunity but shrinks during adolescence

2. Body organ that produces important enzymes for food digestion

3. Largest body organ that is visible to the naked eye

4. Body organ that cleans toxins and metabolizes nutrients/medications

Other Notes:

Daily Logs

Day: _____ Date: _____

VITAL SIGNS

A.M.

Weight: _____ lbs. / kg.
Blood Pressure: _____
Heart Rate: _____ bpm
Oxygen Sat: _____ %
Temperature: _____ F / C

P.M.

Weight: _____ lbs. / kg.
Blood Pressure: _____
Heart Rate: _____ bpm
Oxygen Sat: _____ %
Temperature: _____ F / C

LABORATORY VALUES

WBC: _____
Neutrophils: _____
Hemoglobin: _____
Platelets: _____
Potassium: _____
Calcium: _____
Magnesium: _____
Creatinine: _____
Glucose: _____
ALT: _____
AST: _____
Other (   ): _____

SYMPTOMS EXPERIENCED

Nausea	Y/N	Abdominal Pain	Y/N
Vomiting	Y/N	Shortness of Breath	Y/N
Dizziness	Y/N	Chest Pain	Y/N
Diarrhea	Y/N	Heart Palpitations	Y/N
Loose Stools	Y/N	Headache	Y/N
Mouth Sores	Y/N	Acid Reflux/Heartburn	Y/N
Tired/Fatigued	Y/N	Rash	Y/N

TIC-TAC-TOE

Other Notes:
_____
_____
_____
_____
_____
_____
_____
_____
_____

DAILY LOGS

Day: _____   Date: _____

VITAL SIGNS

A.M.

Weight: _____ lbs. / kg.
Blood Pressure: _____
Heart Rate: _____ bpm
Oxygen Sat: _____ %
Temperature: _____ F / C

P.M.

Weight: _____ lbs. / kg.
Blood Pressure: _____
Heart Rate: _____ bpm
Oxygen Sat: _____ %
Temperature: _____ F / C

LABORATORY VALUES

WBC: _____
Neutrophils: _____
Hemoglobin: _____
Platelets: _____
Potassium: _____
Calcium: _____
Magnesium: _____
Creatinine: _____
Glucose: _____
ALT: _____
AST: _____
Other ( ): _____

SYMPTOMS EXPERIENCED

Nausea	Y/N	Abdominal Pain	Y/N
Vomiting	Y/N	Shortness of Breath	Y/N
Dizziness	Y/N	Chest Pain	Y/N
Diarrhea	Y/N	Heart Palpitations	Y/N
Loose Stools	Y/N	Headache	Y/N
Mouth Sores	Y/N	Acid Reflux/Heartburn	Y/N
Tired/Fatigued	Y/N	Rash	Y/N

Daily Logs

	1	3	
	2		
	4		
2	3		4

Other Notes:
_____
_____
_____
_____
_____
_____
_____
_____

Daily Logs

Day: _____   Date: _____

VITAL SIGNS

A.M.

Weight: _____ lbs. / kg.
Blood Pressure: _____
Heart Rate: _____ bpm
Oxygen Sat: _____ %
Temperature: _____ F / C

P.M.

Weight: _____ lbs. / kg.
Blood Pressure: _____
Heart Rate: _____ bpm
Oxygen Sat: _____ %
Temperature: _____ F / C

LABORATORY VALUES

WBC: _____
Neutrophils: _____
Hemoglobin: _____
Platelets: _____
Potassium: _____
Calcium: _____
Magnesium: _____
Creatinine: _____
Glucose: _____
ALT: _____
AST: _____
Other ( ): _____

SYMPTOMS EXPERIENCED

Nausea	Y/N	Abdominal Pain	Y/N
Vomiting	Y/N	Shortness of Breath	Y/N
Dizziness	Y/N	Chest Pain	Y/N
Diarrhea	Y/N	Heart Palpitations	Y/N
Loose Stools	Y/N	Headache	Y/N
Mouth Sores	Y/N	Acid Reflux/Heartburn	Y/N
Tired/Fatigued	Y/N	Rash	Y/N

Daily Logs

A	O	M	U	X	A	G	W	Z	S
L	H	Q	S	T	T	C	U	R	C
E	L	O	H	T	C	L	T	U	K
I	E	E	G	Z	E	N	Y	Z	C
F	C	A	J	L	A	F	E	N	L
W	A	O	T	H	I	V	K	Y	N
C	T	R	P	B	X	D	A	Z	U
N	U	E	D	U	C	K	N	J	W
T	L	U	J	B	L	F	S	S	A
E	D	O	L	P	H	I	N	Z	B

SNAKE   ELEPHANT   CAT

TURTLE   DOLPHIN   DUCK

Other Notes:
_____
_____
_____
_____
_____

Daily Logs

Day: _____   Date: _____

VITAL SIGNS

A.M.

Weight: _____ lbs. / kg.
Blood Pressure: _____
Heart Rate: _____ bpm
Oxygen Sat: _____ %
Temperature: _____ F / C

P.M.

Weight: _____ lbs. / kg.
Blood Pressure: _____
Heart Rate: _____ bpm
Oxygen Sat: _____ %
Temperature: _____ F / C

LABORATORY VALUES

WBC: _____
Neutrophils: _____
Hemoglobin: _____
Platelets: _____
Potassium: _____
Calcium: _____
Magnesium: _____
Creatinine: _____
Glucose: _____
ALT: _____
AST: _____
Other ( ): _____

SYMPTOMS EXPERIENCED

Nausea	Y/N	Abdominal Pain	Y/N
Vomiting	Y/N	Shortness of Breath	Y/N
Dizziness	Y/N	Chest Pain	Y/N
Diarrhea	Y/N	Heart Palpitations	Y/N
Loose Stools	Y/N	Headache	Y/N
Mouth Sores	Y/N	Acid Reflux/Heartburn	Y/N
Tired/Fatigued	Y/N	Rash	Y/N

FALL SEASON

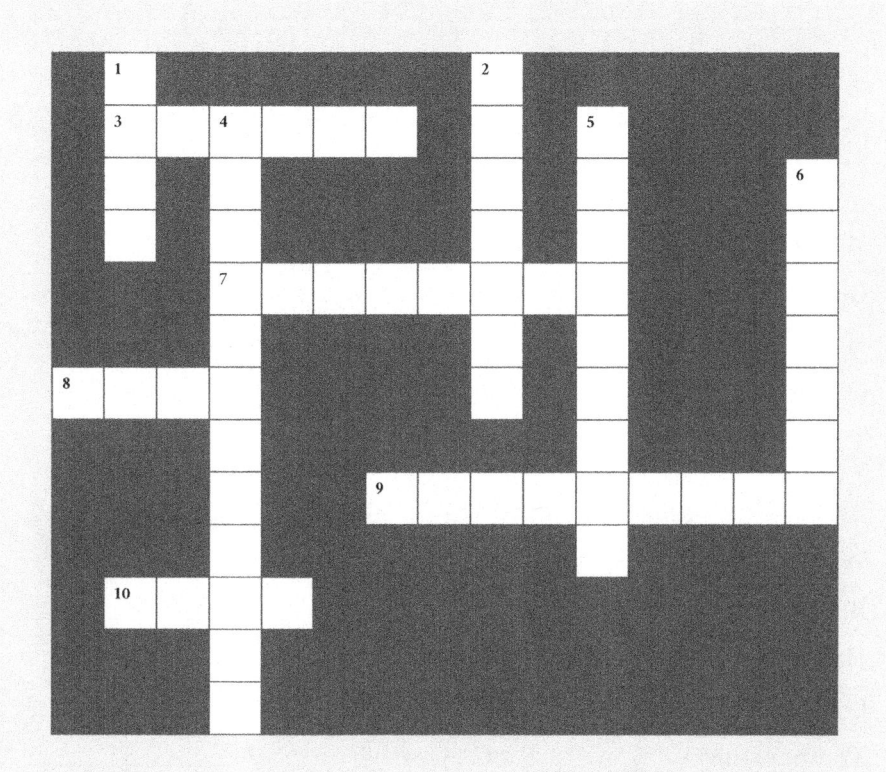

ACROSS:
3. Another word for the fall season
7. The eleventh month of the year
8. What squirrels often gather
9. October 31st
10. Semi-frozen rain

DOWN:
1. The season that follows Summer
2. The tenth month of the year
4. The fourth Thursday in November
5. Used to keep birds off crops
6. Common Halloween decoration

Other Notes:

Daily Logs

Day: _____ Date: _____

VITAL SIGNS

A.M.

Weight: _____ lbs. / kg.
Blood Pressure: _____
Heart Rate: _____ bpm
Oxygen Sat: _____ %
Temperature: _____ F / C

P.M.

Weight: _____ lbs. / kg.
Blood Pressure: _____
Heart Rate: _____ bpm
Oxygen Sat: _____ %
Temperature: _____ F / C

LABORATORY VALUES

WBC: _____
Neutrophils: _____
Hemoglobin: _____
Platelets: _____
Potassium: _____
Calcium: _____
Magnesium: _____
Creatinine: _____
Glucose: _____
ALT: _____
AST: _____
Other ( ): _____

SYMPTOMS EXPERIENCED

Nausea	Y/N	Abdominal Pain	Y/N
Vomiting	Y/N	Shortness of Breath	Y/N
Dizziness	Y/N	Chest Pain	Y/N
Diarrhea	Y/N	Heart Palpitations	Y/N
Loose Stools	Y/N	Headache	Y/N
Mouth Sores	Y/N	Acid Reflux/Heartburn	Y/N
Tired/Fatigued	Y/N	Rash	Y/N

Daily Logs

TIC-TAC-TOE

Other Notes:
_____
_____
_____
_____
_____
_____
_____
_____
_____
_____

Daily Logs

Day: _____ Date: _____

VITAL SIGNS

A.M.

Weight: _____ lbs. / kg.
Blood Pressure: _____
Heart Rate: _____ bpm
Oxygen Sat: _____ %
Temperature: _____ F / C

P.M.

Weight: _____ lbs. / kg.
Blood Pressure: _____
Heart Rate: _____ bpm
Oxygen Sat: _____ %
Temperature: _____ F / C

LABORATORY VALUES

WBC: _____
Neutrophils: _____
Hemoglobin: _____
Platelets: _____
Potassium: _____
Calcium: _____
Magnesium: _____
Creatinine: _____
Glucose: _____
ALT: _____
AST: _____
Other ( ): _____

SYMPTOMS EXPERIENCED

Nausea	Y/N	Abdominal Pain	Y/N
Vomiting	Y/N	Shortness of Breath	Y/N
Dizziness	Y/N	Chest Pain	Y/N
Diarrhea	Y/N	Heart Palpitations	Y/N
Loose Stools	Y/N	Headache	Y/N
Mouth Sores	Y/N	Acid Reflux/Heartburn	Y/N
Tired/Fatigued	Y/N	Rash	Y/N

Daily Logs

	2	3	1	6	5
		6	4	3	
				4	
2		4	3		6
6	4				3
5		2			4

Other Notes:
_____
_____
_____
_____
_____
_____
_____
_____
_____
_____

Daily Logs

Day: _____   Date: _____

VITAL SIGNS

A.M.

Weight: _____ lbs. / kg.
Blood Pressure: _____
Heart Rate: _____ bpm
Oxygen Sat: _____ %
Temperature: _____ F / C

P.M.

Weight: _____ lbs. / kg.
Blood Pressure: _____
Heart Rate: _____ bpm
Oxygen Sat: _____ %
Temperature: _____ F / C

LABORATORY VALUES

WBC: _____
Neutrophils: _____
Hemoglobin: _____
Platelets: _____
Potassium: _____
Calcium: _____
Magnesium: _____
Creatinine: _____
Glucose: _____
ALT: _____
AST: _____
Other ( ): _____

SYMPTOMS EXPERIENCED

Nausea	Y/N	Abdominal Pain	Y/N
Vomiting	Y/N	Shortness of Breath	Y/N
Dizziness	Y/N	Chest Pain	Y/N
Diarrhea	Y/N	Heart Palpitations	Y/N
Loose Stools	Y/N	Headache	Y/N
Mouth Sores	Y/N	Acid Reflux/Heartburn	Y/N
Tired/Fatigued	Y/N	Rash	Y/N

Daily Logs

```
D  B  A  S  E  B  A  L  L  Y  O  J
C  O  O  K  I  N  G  J  I  S  S  J
F  P  X  Y  G  N  I  C  N  A  D  T
H  N  G  N  I  F  R  U  S  B  D  N
K  I  S  O  G  N  I  T  T  I  N  K
V  P  K  W  P  D  W  Y  L  K  Z  M
R  C  X  I  V  G  N  I  G  N  I  S
R  D  Y  E  N  U  N  J  W  T  I  Y
N  R  N  S  B  G  I  A  E  M  O  E
A  K  O  Q  S  S  E  H  C  F  Q  F
X  V  G  N  I  P  P  O  H  S  Y  R
B  Q  N  O  I  T  A  T  I  D  E  M
```

DANCING   **SINGING**   **HIKING**   **SHOPPING**

SURFING   **COOKING**   **KNITTING**   **CHESS**

MEDITATION   **BASEBALL**

Other Notes:
_____
_____
_____
_____

Daily Logs

Day: _____   Date: _____

VITAL SIGNS

A.M.

Weight: _____ lbs. / kg.
Blood Pressure: _____
Heart Rate: _____ bpm
Oxygen Sat: _____ %
Temperature: _____ F / C

P.M.

Weight: _____ lbs. / kg.
Blood Pressure: _____
Heart Rate: _____ bpm
Oxygen Sat: _____ %
Temperature: _____ F / C

LABORATORY VALUES

WBC: _____
Neutrophils: _____
Hemoglobin: _____
Platelets: _____
Potassium: _____
Calcium: _____
Magnesium: _____
Creatinine: _____
Glucose: _____
ALT: _____
AST: _____
Other ( ): _____

SYMPTOMS EXPERIENCED

Nausea	Y/N	Abdominal Pain	Y/N
Vomiting	Y/N	Shortness of Breath	Y/N
Dizziness	Y/N	Chest Pain	Y/N
Diarrhea	Y/N	Heart Palpitations	Y/N
Loose Stools	Y/N	Headache	Y/N
Mouth Sores	Y/N	Acid Reflux/Heartburn	Y/N
Tired/Fatigued	Y/N	Rash	Y/N

CHRISTMAS SEASON

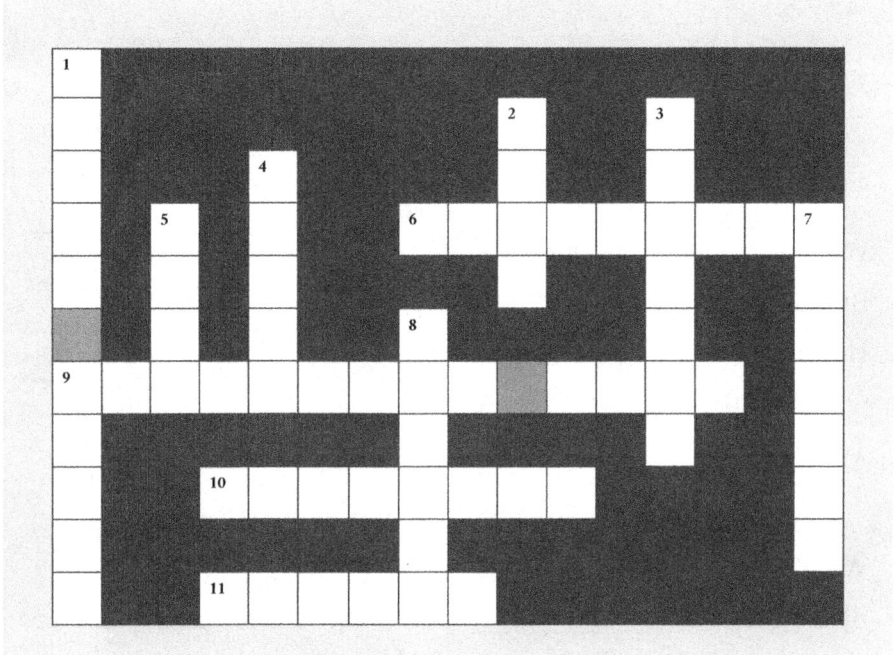

ACROSS:
6. You can fill it with candy, small toys, and gifts
9. People have it in their home and like to decorate it *(2 words)*
10. They pull Santa's sleigh
11. In what season is Christmas day

DOWN:
1. He brings children their presents on Christmas day *(2 words)*
2. It's cold and white
3. Santa Claus comes through it
4. Santa's helpers
5. On January 1st we say "Happy New..."
7. Looks like a man made of snow
8. Light made of wax

Other Notes:

Daily Logs

Day: _____   Date: _____

VITAL SIGNS

A.M.

Weight: _____ lbs. / kg.
Blood Pressure: _____
Heart Rate: _____ bpm
Oxygen Sat: _____ %
Temperature: _____ F / C

P.M.

Weight: _____ lbs. / kg.
Blood Pressure: _____
Heart Rate: _____ bpm
Oxygen Sat: _____ %
Temperature: _____ F / C

LABORATORY VALUES

WBC: _____
Neutrophils: _____
Hemoglobin: _____
Platelets: _____
Potassium: _____
Calcium: _____
Magnesium: _____
Creatinine: _____
Glucose: _____
ALT: _____
AST: _____
Other (_____): _____

SYMPTOMS EXPERIENCED

Nausea	Y/N	Abdominal Pain	Y/N
Vomiting	Y/N	Shortness of Breath	Y/N
Dizziness	Y/N	Chest Pain	Y/N
Diarrhea	Y/N	Heart Palpitations	Y/N
Loose Stools	Y/N	Headache	Y/N
Mouth Sores	Y/N	Acid Reflux/Heartburn	Y/N
Tired/Fatigued	Y/N	Rash	Y/N

Daily Logs

TIC-TAC-TOE

Other Notes:

Daily Logs

Day: _____   Date: _____

VITAL SIGNS

A.M.

Weight: _____ lbs. / kg.
Blood Pressure: _____
Heart Rate: _____ bpm
Oxygen Sat: _____ %
Temperature: _____ F / C

P.M.

Weight: _____ lbs. / kg.
Blood Pressure: _____
Heart Rate: _____ bpm
Oxygen Sat: _____ %
Temperature: _____ F / C

LABORATORY VALUES

WBC: _____
Neutrophils: _____
Hemoglobin: _____
Platelets: _____
Potassium: _____
Calcium: _____
Magnesium: _____
Creatinine: _____
Glucose: _____
ALT: _____
AST: _____
Other (   ): _____

SYMPTOMS EXPERIENCED

Nausea	Y/N	Abdominal Pain	Y/N
Vomiting	Y/N	Shortness of Breath	Y/N
Dizziness	Y/N	Chest Pain	Y/N
Diarrhea	Y/N	Heart Palpitations	Y/N
Loose Stools	Y/N	Headache	Y/N
Mouth Sores	Y/N	Acid Reflux/Heartburn	Y/N
Tired/Fatigued	Y/N	Rash	Y/N

Daily Logs

	4	2		5	1
3				2	
			2	1	
	3		5	4	6
	2				5
		6	1		2

Other Notes:
_____
_____
_____
_____
_____
_____
_____
_____
_____
_____

Daily Logs

Day: _____ Date: _____

VITAL SIGNS

A.M.

Weight: _____ lbs. / kg.
Blood Pressure: _____
Heart Rate: _____ bpm
Oxygen Sat: _____ %
Temperature: _____ F / C

P.M.

Weight: _____ lbs. / kg.
Blood Pressure: _____
Heart Rate: _____ bpm
Oxygen Sat: _____ %
Temperature: _____ F / C

LABORATORY VALUES

WBC: _____
Neutrophils: _____
Hemoglobin: _____
Platelets: _____
Potassium: _____
Calcium: _____
Magnesium: _____
Creatinine: _____
Glucose: _____
ALT: _____
AST: _____
Other ( ): _____

SYMPTOMS EXPERIENCED

Nausea	Y/N	Abdominal Pain	Y/N
Vomiting	Y/N	Shortness of Breath	Y/N
Dizziness	Y/N	Chest Pain	Y/N
Diarrhea	Y/N	Heart Palpitations	Y/N
Loose Stools	Y/N	Headache	Y/N
Mouth Sores	Y/N	Acid Reflux/Heartburn	Y/N
Tired/Fatigued	Y/N	Rash	Y/N

Daily Logs

X	B	I	R	O	N	I	N	G	W	Y	D
A	F	O	X	M	O	P	P	I	N	G	U
X	L	R	F	O	L	D	I	N	G	G	S
G	O	G	W	A	L	K	I	N	G	N	T
N	S	A	C	R	I	B	V	C	G	G	I
I	S	N	N	A	I	I	M	N	N	G	N
V	I	I	I	Q	T	R	I	I	N	X	G
I	N	Z	L	W	H	P	H	I	R	O	U
R	G	I	S	J	E	T	T	J	X	Q	C
D	O	N	H	E	A	A	U	Z	M	P	M
D	U	G	W	B	E	S	M	G	I	D	V
F	A	S	G	N	I	N	A	E	L	C	M

IRONING **BATHING** **SWEEPING** **DUSTING**
ORGANIZING **MOPPING** **WALKING** **DRIVING**
FOLDING **CLEANING** **FLOSSING** **EATING**

Other Notes:
_____
_____
_____
_____

Daily Logs

Day: _____   Date: _____

VITAL SIGNS

A.M.

Weight: _____ lbs. / kg.
Blood Pressure: _____
Heart Rate: _____ bpm
Oxygen Sat: _____ %
Temperature: _____ F / C

P.M.

Weight: _____ lbs. / kg.
Blood Pressure: _____
Heart Rate: _____ bpm
Oxygen Sat: _____ %
Temperature: _____ F / C

LABORATORY VALUES

WBC: _____
Neutrophils: _____
Hemoglobin: _____
Platelets: _____
Potassium: _____
Calcium: _____
Magnesium: _____
Creatinine: _____
Glucose: _____
ALT: _____
AST: _____
Other (_____): _____

SYMPTOMS EXPERIENCED

Nausea	Y/N	Abdominal Pain	Y/N
Vomiting	Y/N	Shortness of Breath	Y/N
Dizziness	Y/N	Chest Pain	Y/N
Diarrhea	Y/N	Heart Palpitations	Y/N
Loose Stools	Y/N	Headache	Y/N
Mouth Sores	Y/N	Acid Reflux/Heartburn	Y/N
Tired/Fatigued	Y/N	Rash	Y/N

Daily Logs

SPORTS

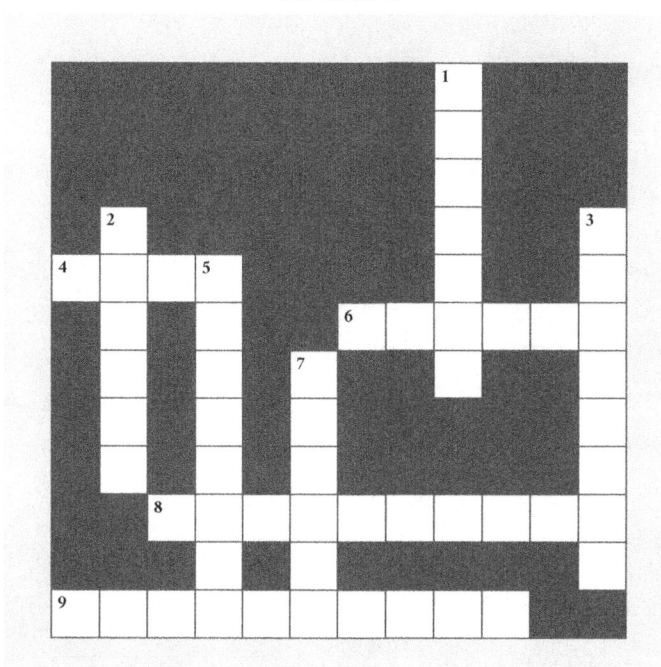

ACROSS:

4. Played outside where players hit a small white ball with a club

6. Played with a racket and yellow ball that palyers hit over a net

8. Played with 10 players on the court. Players can shoot the ball into the hoop

9. Can be played on the beach where players hit a ball over a net

DOWN:

1. Played by throwing a ball down an alley. If you hit down all ten pins you get a strike

2. Played on a large open field where players can only use their feet to kick the ball into a goal

3. Played on a diamond shaped field where players run the base and score homeruns

5. Has many players on the field and on the sideline. They score touchdowns and kick fieldgoals

7. Played on the ice and the players use sticks to hit the puck into the goal

Other Notes:

Daily Logs

Day: _____ Date: _____

VITAL SIGNS

A.M.

Weight: _____ lbs. / kg.
Blood Pressure: _____
Heart Rate: _____ bpm
Oxygen Sat: _____ %
Temperature: _____ F / C

P.M.

Weight: _____ lbs. / kg.
Blood Pressure: _____
Heart Rate: _____ bpm
Oxygen Sat: _____ %
Temperature: _____ F / C

LABORATORY VALUES

WBC: _____
Neutrophils: _____
Hemoglobin: _____
Platelets: _____
Potassium: _____
Calcium: _____
Magnesium: _____
Creatinine: _____
Glucose: _____
ALT: _____
AST: _____
Other ( ): _____

SYMPTOMS EXPERIENCED

Nausea	Y/N	Abdominal Pain	Y/N
Vomiting	Y/N	Shortness of Breath	Y/N
Dizziness	Y/N	Chest Pain	Y/N
Diarrhea	Y/N	Heart Palpitations	Y/N
Loose Stools	Y/N	Headache	Y/N
Mouth Sores	Y/N	Acid Reflux/Heartburn	Y/N
Tired/Fatigued	Y/N	Rash	Y/N

TIC-TAC-TOE

Other Notes:

Daily Logs

Day: _____   Date: _____

VITAL SIGNS

A.M.

Weight: _____ lbs. / kg.
Blood Pressure: _____
Heart Rate: _____ bpm
Oxygen Sat: _____ %
Temperature: _____ F / C

P.M.

Weight: _____ lbs. / kg.
Blood Pressure: _____
Heart Rate: _____ bpm
Oxygen Sat: _____ %
Temperature: _____ F / C

LABORATORY VALUES

WBC: _____
Neutrophils: _____
Hemoglobin: _____
Platelets: _____
Potassium: _____
Calcium: _____
Magnesium: _____
Creatinine: _____
Glucose: _____
ALT: _____
AST: _____
Other ( ): _____

SYMPTOMS EXPERIENCED

Nausea	Y/N	Abdominal Pain	Y/N
Vomiting	Y/N	Shortness of Breath	Y/N
Dizziness	Y/N	Chest Pain	Y/N
Diarrhea	Y/N	Heart Palpitations	Y/N
Loose Stools	Y/N	Headache	Y/N
Mouth Sores	Y/N	Acid Reflux/Heartburn	Y/N
Tired/Fatigued	Y/N	Rash	Y/N

Daily Logs

6				5	
	2	5			1
3		6	1		5
1		2		4	
2		1			
5					

Other Notes:

_____
_____
_____
_____
_____
_____
_____
_____
_____
_____

Daily Logs

Day: _____   Date: _____

VITAL SIGNS

A.M.

Weight: _____ lbs. / kg.
Blood Pressure: _____
Heart Rate: _____ bpm
Oxygen Sat: _____ %
Temperature: _____ F / C

P.M.

Weight: _____ lbs. / kg.
Blood Pressure: _____
Heart Rate: _____ bpm
Oxygen Sat: _____ %
Temperature: _____ F / C

LABORATORY VALUES

WBC: _____
Neutrophils: _____
Hemoglobin: _____
Platelets: _____
Potassium: _____
Calcium: _____
Magnesium: _____
Creatinine: _____
Glucose: _____
ALT: _____
AST: _____
Other ( ): _____

SYMPTOMS EXPERIENCED

Nausea	Y/N	Abdominal Pain	Y/N
Vomiting	Y/N	Shortness of Breath	Y/N
Dizziness	Y/N	Chest Pain	Y/N
Diarrhea	Y/N	Heart Palpitations	Y/N
Loose Stools	Y/N	Headache	Y/N
Mouth Sores	Y/N	Acid Reflux/Heartburn	Y/N
Tired/Fatigued	Y/N	Rash	Y/N

Daily Logs

S	W	E	A	T	E	R	T	A	N
I	V	G	S	O	C	K	S	G	R
E	T	W	S	T	F	F	U	E	T
C	R	E	E	S	R	A	S	U	E
A	L	M	O	S	E	H	T	V	L
L	C	U	H	Y	I	V	A	A	E
K	E	F	S	R	V	X	T	D	C
C	I	R	T	V	O	G	F	N	A
E	T	E	W	A	T	C	H	V	R
N	F	P	W	S	T	N	A	P	B

PERFUME   **SHOES**   **NECKLACE**

PANTS   **SHIRT**   **BRACELET**

SOCKS   **TIE**   **WATCH**   **SWEATER**

Other Notes:
_____
_____
_____
_____
_____

Daily Logs

Day:	Date:

VITAL SIGNS

A.M.

Weight: _____ lbs. / kg.
Blood Pressure: _____
Heart Rate: _____ bpm
Oxygen Sat: _____ %
Temperature: _____ F / C

P.M.

Weight: _____ lbs. / kg.
Blood Pressure: _____
Heart Rate: _____ bpm
Oxygen Sat: _____ %
Temperature: _____ F / C

LABORATORY VALUES

WBC: _____
Neutrophils: _____
Hemoglobin: _____
Platelets: _____
Potassium: _____
Calcium: _____
Magnesium: _____
Creatinine: _____
Glucose: _____
ALT: _____
AST: _____
Other ( ): _____

SYMPTOMS EXPERIENCED

Nausea	Y/N	Abdominal Pain	Y/N
Vomiting	Y/N	Shortness of Breath	Y/N
Dizziness	Y/N	Chest Pain	Y/N
Diarrhea	Y/N	Heart Palpitations	Y/N
Loose Stools	Y/N	Headache	Y/N
Mouth Sores	Y/N	Acid Reflux/Heartburn	Y/N
Tired/Fatigued	Y/N	Rash	Y/N

FAST FOOD

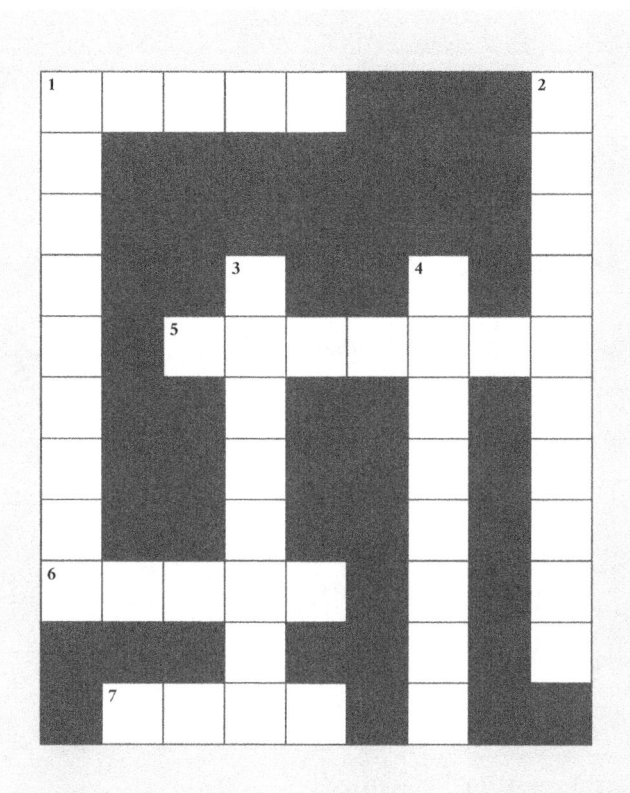

ACROSS:
1. Italin pie with toppings
5. Small chicken pieces
6. Tube used to drink with
7. Fizzy drink

DOWN:
1. Knot shaped breads
2. Frozen milk dessert
3. Yellow condiment
4. Condiment made with tomatoes

Other Notes:

Daily Logs

Day: _____   Date: _____

VITAL SIGNS

A.M.

Weight: _____ lbs. / kg.
Blood Pressure: _____
Heart Rate: _____ bpm
Oxygen Sat: _____ %
Temperature: _____ F / C

P.M.

Weight: _____ lbs. / kg.
Blood Pressure: _____
Heart Rate: _____ bpm
Oxygen Sat: _____ %
Temperature: _____ F / C

LABORATORY VALUES

WBC: _____
Neutrophils: _____
Hemoglobin: _____
Platelets: _____
Potassium: _____
Calcium: _____
Magnesium: _____
Creatinine: _____
Glucose: _____
ALT: _____
AST: _____
Other ( ): _____

SYMPTOMS EXPERIENCED

Nausea	Y/N	Abdominal Pain	Y/N
Vomiting	Y/N	Shortness of Breath	Y/N
Dizziness	Y/N	Chest Pain	Y/N
Diarrhea	Y/N	Heart Palpitations	Y/N
Loose Stools	Y/N	Headache	Y/N
Mouth Sores	Y/N	Acid Reflux/Heartburn	Y/N
Tired/Fatigued	Y/N	Rash	Y/N

TIC-TAC-TOE

Other Notes:

DAILY LOGS

Day: _____   Date: _____

VITAL SIGNS

A.M.

Weight: _____ lbs. / kg.
Blood Pressure: _____
Heart Rate: _____ bpm
Oxygen Sat: _____ %
Temperature: _____ F / C

P.M.

Weight: _____ lbs. / kg.
Blood Pressure: _____
Heart Rate: _____ bpm
Oxygen Sat: _____ %
Temperature: _____ F / C

LABORATORY VALUES

WBC: _____
Neutrophils: _____
Hemoglobin: _____
Platelets: _____
Potassium: _____
Calcium: _____
Magnesium: _____
Creatinine: _____
Glucose: _____
ALT: _____
AST: _____
Other (__): _____

SYMPTOMS EXPERIENCED

Nausea	Y/N	Abdominal Pain	Y/N
Vomiting	Y/N	Shortness of Breath	Y/N
Dizziness	Y/N	Chest Pain	Y/N
Diarrhea	Y/N	Heart Palpitations	Y/N
Loose Stools	Y/N	Headache	Y/N
Mouth Sores	Y/N	Acid Reflux/Heartburn	Y/N
Tired/Fatigued	Y/N	Rash	Y/N

Daily Logs

8	4	6	9	5		2		7
2		5		1	4			8
9	1	3		2			5	6
1	5		7	6	9		2	4
6				4	1	8	7	
7	3	4	2	8	5			
		1	4	9	2		8	
4	8						9	2
	9	2	5	7				

Other Notes:

Daily Logs

Day: _____ Date: _____

VITAL SIGNS

A.M.

Weight: _____ lbs. / kg.
Blood Pressure: _____
Heart Rate: _____ bpm
Oxygen Sat: _____ %
Temperature: _____ F / C

P.M.

Weight: _____ lbs. / kg.
Blood Pressure: _____
Heart Rate: _____ bpm
Oxygen Sat: _____ %
Temperature: _____ F / C

LABORATORY VALUES

WBC: _____
Neutrophils: _____
Hemoglobin: _____
Platelets: _____
Potassium: _____
Calcium: _____
Magnesium: _____
Creatinine: _____
Glucose: _____
ALT: _____
AST: _____
Other ( ): _____

SYMPTOMS EXPERIENCED

Nausea	Y/N	Abdominal Pain	Y/N
Vomiting	Y/N	Shortness of Breath	Y/N
Dizziness	Y/N	Chest Pain	Y/N
Diarrhea	Y/N	Heart Palpitations	Y/N
Loose Stools	Y/N	Headache	Y/N
Mouth Sores	Y/N	Acid Reflux/Heartburn	Y/N
Tired/Fatigued	Y/N	Rash	Y/N

Daily Logs

W	S	T	A	R	F	I	S	H	T	X
S	H	A	K	E	W	H	A	L	E	I
U	A	P	L	A	E	S	H	S	S	O
E	C	R	A	B	G	I	J	T	A	K
S	G	B	O	U	F	M	N	B	I	Z
R	I	L	O	B	S	T	E	R	V	T
O	A	O	C	T	O	P	U	S	V	U
H	X	V	N	I	H	P	L	O	D	N
A	J	E	L	L	Y	F	I	S	H	A
E	Z	I	E	L	T	R	U	T	K	W
S	G	Y	Y	H	C	P	T	R	M	W

SEAL	DOLPHIN	WHALE	STARFISH
LOBSTER	TURTLE	OCTOPUS	JELLYFISH
SHARK	CRAB	TUNA	SEAHORSE

Other Notes:

_____
_____
_____
_____

Daily Logs

Day: _____   Date: _____

VITAL SIGNS

A.M.
Weight: _____ lbs. / kg.
Blood Pressure: _____
Heart Rate: _____ bpm
Oxygen Sat: _____ %
Temperature: _____ F / C

P.M.
Weight: _____ lbs. / kg.
Blood Pressure: _____
Heart Rate: _____ bpm
Oxygen Sat: _____ %
Temperature: _____ F / C

LABORATORY VALUES

WBC: _____
Neutrophils: _____
Hemoglobin: _____
Platelets: _____
Potassium: _____
Calcium: _____
Magnesium: _____
Creatinine: _____
Glucose: _____
ALT: _____
AST: _____
Other ( ): _____

SYMPTOMS EXPERIENCED

Nausea	Y/N	Abdominal Pain	Y/N
Vomiting	Y/N	Shortness of Breath	Y/N
Dizziness	Y/N	Chest Pain	Y/N
Diarrhea	Y/N	Heart Palpitations	Y/N
Loose Stools	Y/N	Headache	Y/N
Mouth Sores	Y/N	Acid Reflux/Heartburn	Y/N
Tired/Fatigued	Y/N	Rash	Y/N

FAMOUS MOVIES

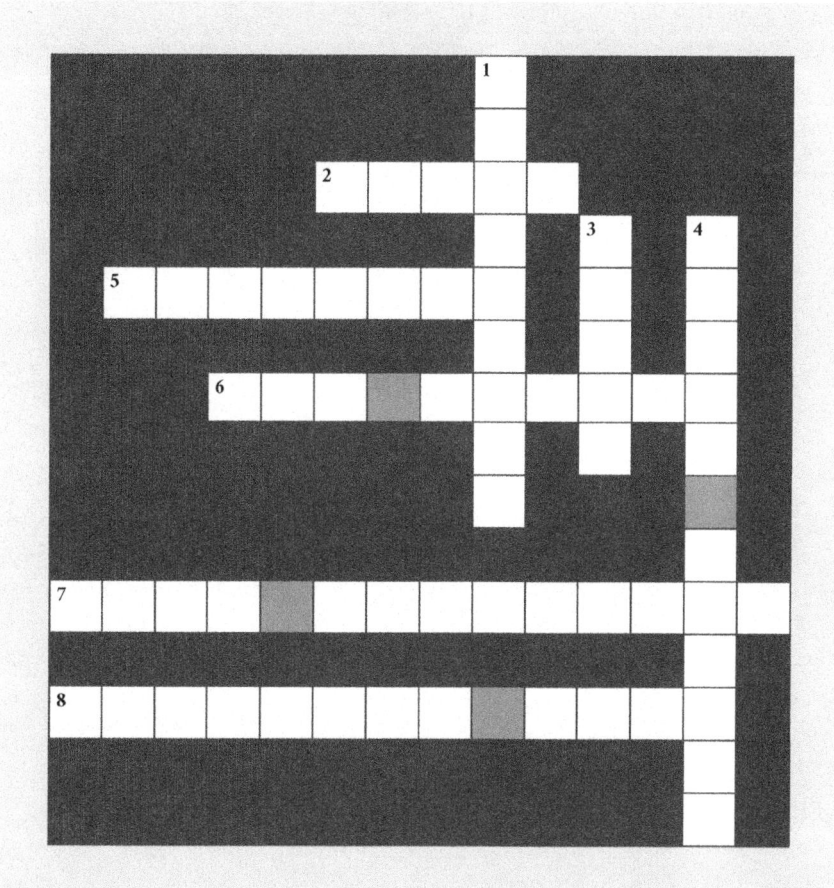

ACROSS:

2. What is the name of the spaceship in the 2008 Pixar film Wall-E

5. What animal is Rango from the 2011 Nickelodeon movie Rango

6. In the Harry Potter films, what is Lord Voldemort's real name

7. The name of the spaceman in Pixar's Toy Story

8. What is the name of the 1993 movie about a safari with dinosaurs

DOWN:

1. In the 2003 Pixar movie Finding Nemo, what type of fish is Nemo

3. In Kung-Fu Panda, what animal is Po

4. What is Spiderman's real name

GLOSSARY

Abdominal pain: Abdominal pain is when your stomach or belly hurts.

Acid reflux: When stomach juices go up into the throat, causing a funny feeling or a small burp-like sensation.

ALT: Alanine Aminotransferase, it is a special substance in the body that helps the liver work properly. It's like a helper that shows if the liver is doing well, might go up if liver is under a lot of stress, such as when drinking too much alcohol or when getting chemotherapy. Normal adult range: 4 to 36 U/L.

Allogenic stem cell transplant: A type of stem cell transplant in which the patient receives stem cells that are not his/her own, but rather from a donor.

Antibiotic: A type of medication that fights bacterial infections. They might directly kill the bacteria or just stop them from multiplying while the body's defenses kill them.

Antifungal: Similar to antibiotics, but they fight fungal infections (caused by fungi) instead

Antiviral: Similar to antibiotics, but they fight viral infections (caused by viruses).

Apheresis Line: An intravenous catheter with two or three tubes (known as ports) that is inserted into a vein, with the tip advanced into the central vasculature near the heart. It is capable of receiving/delivering a greater flow than traditional IV lines or chemotherapy ports.

AST: Aspartate Aminotransferase, another special substance in the body that helps the liver and other organs. Might go up if liver if under a lot of stress, such as when drinking too much alcohol or when getting chemotherapy. Normal adult range: 8 to 32 U/L.

Autologous stem cell transplant: A type of stem cell transplant in which the patient receives his/her own stem cells.

BEAM: A type of conditioning chemotherapy regimen, it includes the drugs Carmustine, Etoposide, Cytarabine, and Melphalan.

Blood culture: A laboratory test. The collected blood is stored for days and monitored to see if bacteria or other organisms are growing in the blood. If positive, it helps to find out which organism is causing the infection and specific medications can be given to kill it.

BU/MEL: A type of conditioning chemotherapy regimen, it includes the drugs Busulfan, and Melphalan.

Calcium: A super important mineral that helps your bones and teeth stay strong. It also helps your muscles work and your heart beat just right. Normal adult range: 8.5 to 10.2 mg/dL.

Cardiologist: A medical doctor that specializes in treating conditions of the cardiovascular system.

CBV: A type of conditioning chemotherapy regimen, it includes the drugs Cyclophosphamide, Carmustine, and Etoposide.

CLV: A type of conditioning chemotherapy regimen, it includes the drugs Cyclophosphamide, Lomustine, and Etoposide.

Conditioning chemotherapy: The high doses of chemotherapy or a combination of chemotherapy and radiation therapy given after stem cells are harvested. The high-dose treatment kills cancer cells, but also eliminates the blood-producing stem cells that are left in your bone marrow. Some common conditioning chemotherapy regimens are **BEAM, BU/MEL, CBV, CLV, LACE, LEAM,** and **MITO/MEL.**

Creatinine: A number from a test that tells us how well your kidneys are working. It's like a little report card for your kidneys. Normal adult range: 0.7 to 1.3 mg/dL.

DMSO (Dimethyl Sulfoxide): A clear agent commonly used as a preservative. Used when storing stem cells to prevent damage to them during freezing.

Fasting: The abstention from eating and sometimes drinking for a period of usually 8 hours at least.

Feces: The material excreted from the anus during a bowel movement.

Glucose: A measurement that shows how much sugar is in your blood. Sugar is like the fuel for your body, and it comes from the food you eat, or might be given to you intravenously. Normal adult range when **fasting**: 70 to 100 mg/dL.

Gut Microbiome: An ecosystem of microbes that live in our intestines. They help us digest certain foods and control harmful bacteria.

Gynecologist: A medical doctor that specializes in treating conditions of the female reproductive system.

Heartburn: The feeling of burning in your chest or throat as a consequence of acid reflux.

Hemoglobin: A measurement that tells us about the amount of a special substance in your blood. This substance is like a delivery truck for oxygen, which is needed by your body's cells to work properly. Normal adult range: Males 13.8 to 17.2 g/dL or Females 12.1 to 15.1 g/dL

Inactivated Vaccine: A vaccine that includes a killed version of a germ that causes a disease, a toxin made by the germ, or only a protein that helps the body generate defenses against a type of germ. Common ones Tdap, Influenza, COVID-19, etc.

Glossary

Influenza: An inactivated vaccine that protects against influenza (flu) viruses. Often recommended yearly.

LACE: A type of conditioning chemotherapy regimen, it includes the drugs Lomustine, Cytarabine, Cyclophosphamide, and Etoposide.

LEAM: A type of conditioning chemotherapy regimen, it includes the drugs Lomustine, Etoposide, Cytarabine, and Melphalan. Magnesium.

Live Vaccine: A vaccine that uses a weakened form of a germ that causes a disease. They create a stronger and longer-lasting immune response, which can provide protection against a germ for a lifetime. Common ones MMR, Varicella, etc.

Lupron (Leuprolide): A man-made hormone injection. It has different uses such as endometriosis, heavy or irregular periods, prostate cancer, among others.

MITO/MEL: A type of conditioning chemotherapy regimen, it includes the drugs Mitoxantrone, and Melphalan.

MMR: A live vaccine that protects against the measles, mumps, and rubella viruses. Often given only during childhood.

Neutrophils: A type of white blood cell, which plays a pivotal role in the body's immune defense mechanism. After a stem cell transplant the number of white blood cells in your body is dramatically reduced. This is called neutropenia. Normal adult range: 2,500 to 8,000 per microliter of blood.

Oxygen Sat: Oxygen saturation refers to the proportion of oxygen-saturated hemoglobin in the bloodstream, typically presented as a percentage. This measurement indicates how effectively the red blood cells are carrying oxygen to different parts of the body. Also called SpO2, Pulse Oximetry, or O2 levels.

PET scan: Short for Positron Emission Tomography. It's a scan that uses radioactive substances to measure and visualize the activity levels of organs. Used commonly to screen for cancer.

Platelets: Platelets are tiny cell fragments that play a vital role in blood clotting and wound healing. Normal adult range: 150,000 to 450,000 per microliter of blood.

Potassium: Potassium is an essential electrolyte that plays a critical role in maintaining proper fluid balance, muscle function, heart function, and nerve signaling in the body. Normal adult range: 3.5 to 5.2 mEq/L.

Preservative Drug: A medication that can be added to food, medications, or cells to prevent or slow down decomposition.

Pulmonologist: A medical doctor that specializes in treating conditions of the respiratory system.

QR code: A Quick Response code is a two-dimensional barcode that contains encoded information. It's like a digital passport that can store a lot of data, such as website links, text, or other details.

Stem cell transplant: A medical procedure that involves replacing damaged or unhealthy cells in the body with healthy stem cells. After preparatory treatments, healthy stem cells are put into the body, helping it produce new and healthy cells.

Stool culture: Similar to a blood culture, but instead of testing blood, human feces are tested for foreign organisms.

Tdap: An inactivated vaccine that protects against tetanus, diphtheria, and pertussis. Often recommended every 10 years.

Varicella: A live vaccine that protects against the varicella-zoster virus (chickenpox). Often given only during childhood.

WBC: A measure of the number of white blood cells in your blood. Normal adult range: 4,000 to 11,000 per microliter of blood.

White Blood Cells: Also known as Leukocytes or WBC. They are cells from the immune system that circulate in the blood and help fight infections and inflammations.

Game Instructions

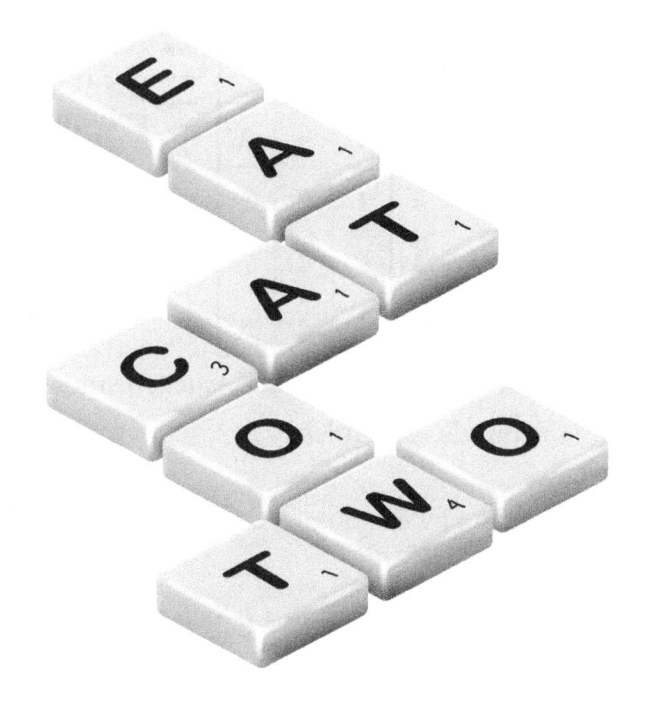

Sudoku

Here is how to solve a traditional 9 by 9 sudoku. Sudoku puzzles require you to find themissing numbers in a 9 by 9 grid, with that grid itself divided into 9 square grids of 3 by 3.

9	8	1	3	6	5	2	7	4
7	6	5	4	8	2	3	1	9
2	4	3	1	7	9	8	5	6
1	9	2	6	3	4	7	8	5
4	3	7	5	2	8	9	6	1
8	5	6	9	1	7	4	3	2
3	2	4	7	5	6	1	9	8
5	1	8	2	9	3	6	4	7
6	7	9	8	4	1	5	2	3

You can't just add any numbers, though. There are rules that make solving the puzzle challenging.

A number can only occur once in a row, column, or square.

To solve a Sudoku, look for open spaces where its row, column, and square already have enough other numbers filled in to tell you the correct value. The more squares you fill in, the easier the puzzle is to finish.

Similarly, in a 4 by 4 sudoku, you can only use the numbers 1, 2, 3, and 4.

Following that same logic, in a 6 by 6 sudoku, you can only use the numbers 1, 2, 3, 4, 5, and 6.

Remember, a number can only occur once in a row, column, or square.

Have fun and exercise your brain.

Game Instructions

Word Search Puzzle

Solving a word search puzzle is easy. You need to find the all the given words that are hidden in the grid.

You might find the words spelled across, up and down, or diagonally. The words might be spelled forward or backward.

See the following sample to give you an idea. On the grid in the right, all of the words have been found already. See how some of the words are spelled backwards, such as Uranus or Earth.

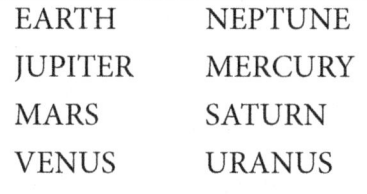

J	S	O	L	U	T	I	S
S	U	N	A	R	U	U	A
N	E	P	T	U	N	E	T
S	O	N	I	E	I	S	U
R	C	E	V	T	R	E	R
A	H	T	R	A	E	S	N
M	M	E	R	C	U	R	Y

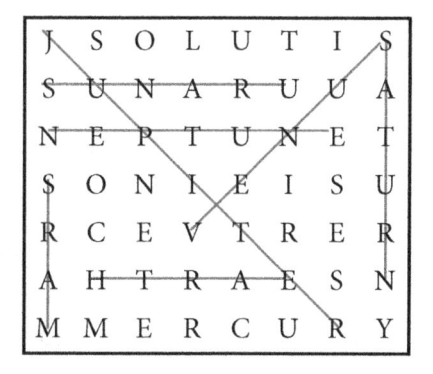

EARTH   NEPTUNE
JUPITER   MERCURY
MARS   SATURN
VENUS   URANUS

Autologous Stem Cell Transplant

Crossword Puzzle

ACROSS:
2. A feline furry animal
4. The ability to understand and share the feelings of another
5. A small brown bird known for chirping

DOWN:
1. A large, four-legged animal is often used for transportation
3. Existing or available in large quantities

Objective:

Enter a correct answer in the crossword puzzle grid for each puzzle clue.

Clues:

- Each across and down clue is assigned a unique number. This number corresponds to the number for its answer in the grid.
- Answers must fit within the allowed space for the clue.
- Words in the crossword puzzle will cross each other, this fact is the source of inspiration for the name of the game.

Game Instructions

How to solve a Crossword Puzzle:

- Select a clue from the across or down list.
- Think up possible answers to the clue.
- Place your answer in the specific numbered white square that corresponds to the clue's type (across or down)
- Continue solving all clues.
- The game ends when every white square is filled in with an answer that the solver believes is correct. That's all there is to it!

Tic-tac-toe

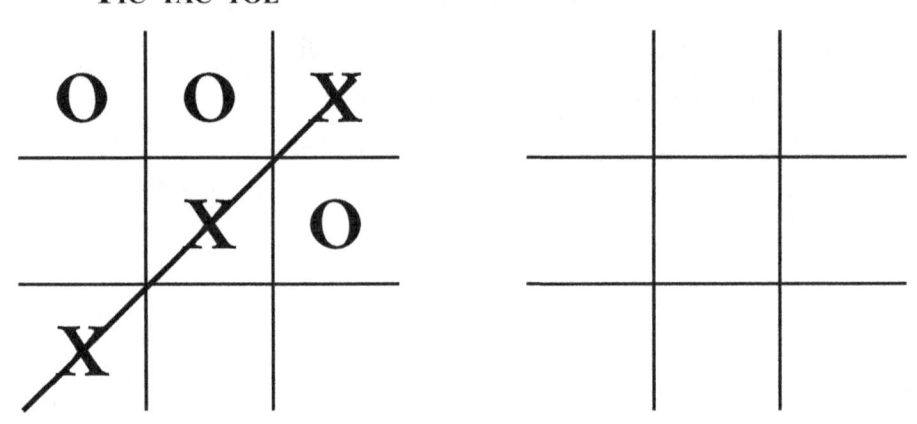

The objective of Tic-tac-toe is to get three in a row, as it can be seen in the example above.

This game is played with two players. The first player is known as X and the second is O. X always goes first.

Players alternate placing Xs and Os on the game board until one of them has three in a row or all nine squares are filled.

Three in a row can be obtained either horizontally, vertically, or diagonally.

Answer Key

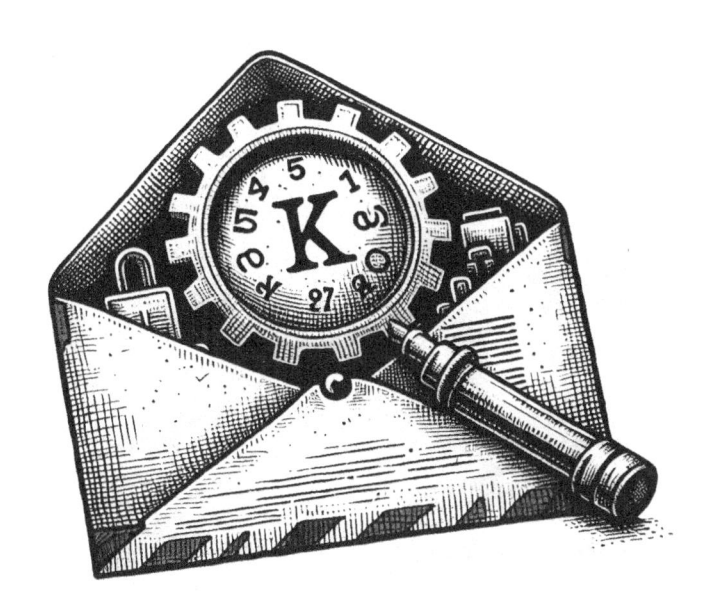

Autologous Stem Cell Transplant

PAGE 41

4	3	1	2
2	1	3	4
3	4	2	1
1	2	4	3

PAGE 43

```
B F U A X L O F I G
G E A S T R N T I B
Z I W E S T D U X S
E Y C N D H M E O N
W B V W D B A U O T
I A H H G L T R K R
M H L R I H T Q T S
I Z K I D H B I B T
D N W R H R W V V D
C M C J N T N E F F
```

EAST WEST NORTH SOUTH

PAGE 45

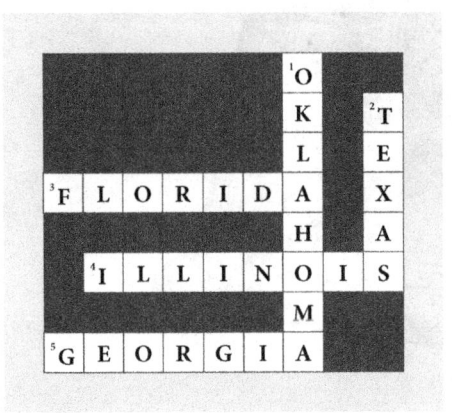

			¹O	
			K	²T
			L	E
³F	L	O	R	I	D	A	X
			H	A
	⁴I	L	L	I	N	O	I	S
			M	
⁵G	E	O	R	G	I	A	

PAGE 49

1	4	2	3
3	2	4	1
2	3	1	4
4	1	3	2

Answer Key

PAGE 51

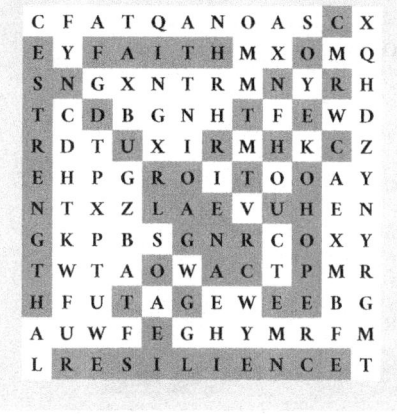

C	F	A	T	Q	A	N	O	A	S	C	X
E	Y	F	A	I	T	H	M	X	O	M	Q
S	N	G	X	N	T	R	M	N	Y	R	H
T	C	D	B	G	N	H	T	F	E	W	D
R	D	T	U	X	I	R	M	H	K	C	Z
E	H	P	G	R	O	I	T	O	O	A	Y
N	T	X	Z	L	A	E	V	U	H	E	N
G	K	P	B	S	G	N	R	C	O	X	Y
T	W	T	A	O	W	A	C	T	P	M	R
H	F	U	T	A	G	E	W	E	E	B	G
A	U	W	F	E	G	H	Y	M	R	F	M
L	R	E	S	I	L	I	E	N	C	E	T

COURAGE ENDURANCE FAITH RESILIENCE
HOPE STRENGTH CONTROL TOGETHER

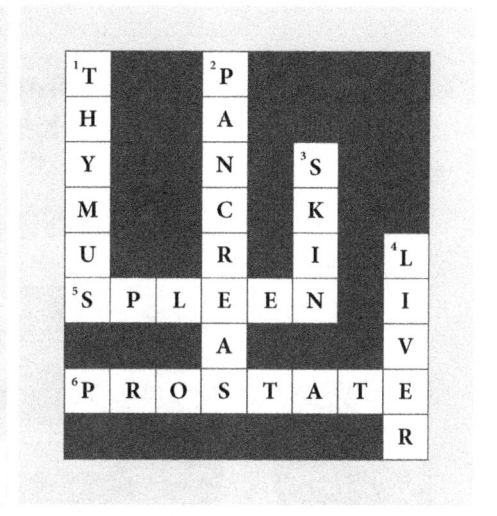

PAGE 53

1 Across: THYMUS
2 Down: PANCREAS
3 Down: SKIN
4 Down: LIVER
5 Across: SPLEEN
6 Across: PROSTATE

PAGE 57

4	1	3	2
3	2	4	1
1	4	2	3
2	3	1	4

PAGE 59

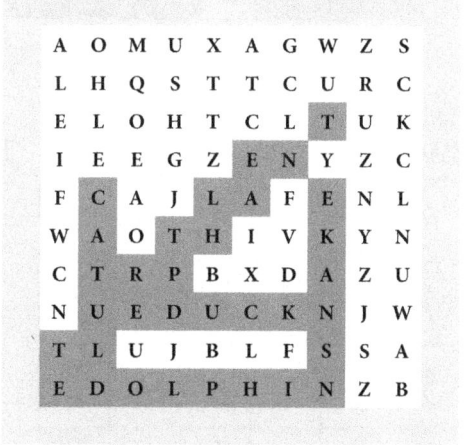

SNAKE ELEPHANT CAT
TURTLE DOLPHIN DUCK

111

Autologous Stem Cell Transplant

PAGE 61

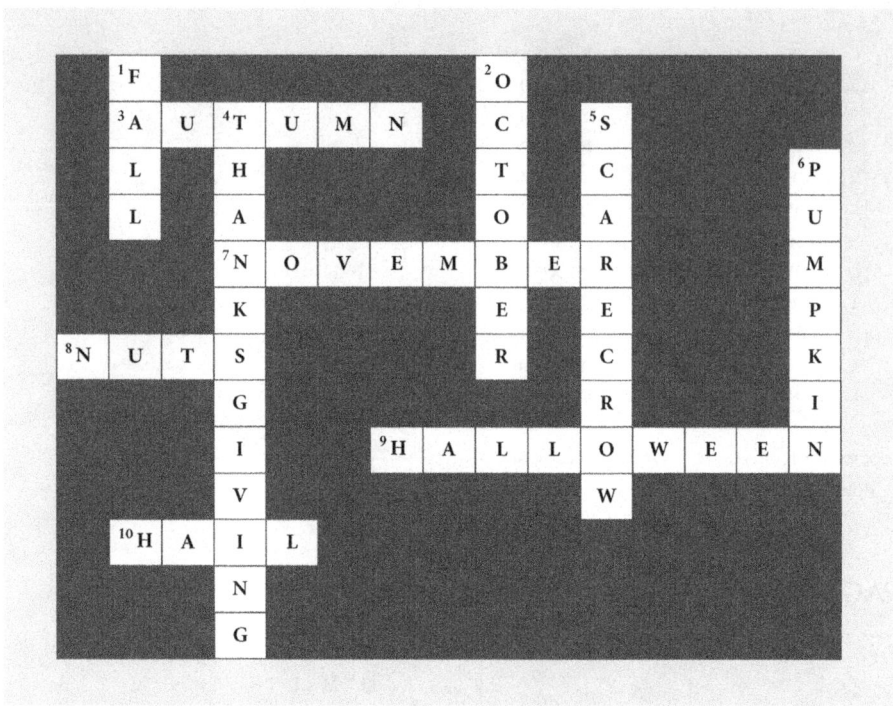

		¹F					²O				
	³A	U	⁴T	U	M	N	C		⁵S		
		L	H				T		C		⁶P
		L	A				O		A		U
			⁷N	O	V	E	M	B	E	R	M
			K				E		E		P
⁸N	U	T	S				R		C		K
			G						R		I
			I		⁹H	A	L	L	O	W	E	E	N
			V						W		
	¹⁰H	A	I	L							
			N								
			G								

PAGE 65

4	2	3	1	6	5
1	5	6	4	3	2
3	6	5	2	4	1
2	1	4	3	5	6
6	4	1	5	2	3
5	3	2	6	1	4

PAGE 67

D	B	A	S	E	B	A	L	L	Y	O	J
C	O	O	K	I	N	G	J	I	S	S	J
F	P	X	Y	G	N	I	C	N	A	D	T
H	N	G	N	I	F	R	U	S	B	D	N
K	I	S	O	G	N	I	T	T	I	N	K
V	P	K	W	P	D	W	Y	L	K	Z	M
R	C	X	I	V	G	N	I	G	N	I	S
R	D	Y	E	N	U	N	J	W	T	I	Y
N	R	N	S	B	G	I	A	E	M	O	E
A	K	O	Q	S	S	E	H	C	F	Q	F
X	V	G	N	I	P	P	O	H	S	Y	R
B	Q	N	O	I	T	A	T	I	D	E	M

DANCING SINGING HIKING SHOPPING
COOKING SURFING CHESS KNITTING
MEDITATION BASEBALL

112

Answer Key

PAGE 69

¹S										
A					²S		³C			
N			⁴E		N		H			
T		⁵Y	L		⁶S	T	O	C	K	I	N	G	⁷S
A		E	V				W		M				N
		A	E		⁸C				N				O
⁹C	H	R	I	S	T	M	A	S		T	R	E	E	W
L					N					Y				M
A			¹⁰R	E	I	N	D	E	E	R				A
U					L									N
S			¹¹W	I	N	T	E	R						

PAGE 73

6	4	2	3	5	1
3	1	5	6	2	4
5	6	4	2	1	3
2	3	1	5	4	6
1	2	3	4	6	5
4	5	6	1	3	2

PAGE 75

MOPPING BATHING DUSTING SWEEPING
ORGANIZING IRONING DRIVING WALKING
CEANING FOLDING EATING FLOSSING

Autologous Stem Cell Transplant

PAGE 77

Crossword solution:
- 1 Down: BOWLING
- 2 Down: SOCCER
- 3 Down: BASEBALL
- 4 Across: GOLF
- 5 Down: FOOTBALL
- 6 Across: TENNIS
- 7 Down: HOCKEY
- 8 Across: BASKETBALL
- 9 Across: VOLLEYBALL

PAGE 81

6	1	3	4	5	2
4	2	5	6	3	1
3	4	6	1	2	5
1	5	2	3	4	6
2	3	1	5	6	4
5	6	4	2	1	3

PAGE 83

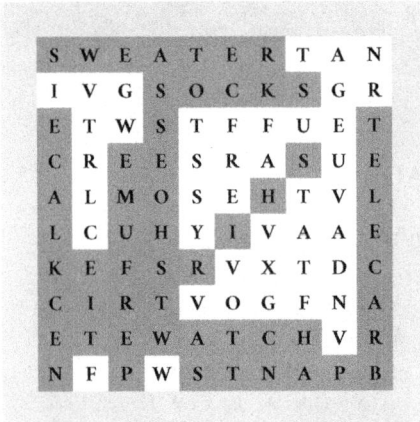

S	W	E	A	T	E	R	T	A	N
I	V	G	S	O	C	K	S	G	R
E	T	W	S	T	F	F	U	E	T
C	R	E	E	S	R	A	S	U	E
A	L	M	O	S	E	H	T	V	L
L	C	U	H	Y	I	V	A	A	E
K	E	F	S	R	V	X	T	D	C
C	I	R	T	V	O	G	F	N	A
E	T	E	W	A	T	C	H	V	R
N	F	P	W	S	T	N	A	P	B

PERFUME SHOES NECKLACE
SWEATER SHIRT BRACELET
SOCKS TIE WATCH PANTS

PAGE 85

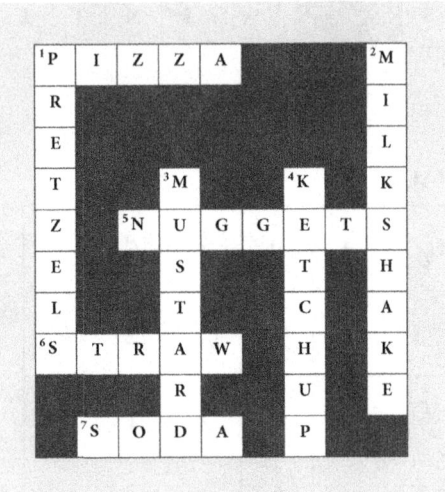

Crossword solution:
- 1 Across: PIZZA
- 1 Down: PRETZEL
- 2 Down: MILKSHAKE
- 3 Down: MUSTARD
- 4 Down: KETCHUP
- 5 Across: NUGGETS
- 6 Across: STRAW
- 7 Across: SODA

114

Answer Key

PAGE 89

8	4	6	9	5	3	2	1	7
2	7	5	6	1	4	9	3	8
9	1	3	8	2	7	4	5	6
1	5	8	7	6	9	3	2	4
6	2	9	3	4	1	8	7	5
7	3	4	2	8	5	1	6	9
5	6	1	4	9	2	7	8	3
4	8	7	1	3	6	5	9	2
3	9	2	5	7	8	6	4	1

PAGE 91

```
W S T A R F I S H T X
S H A K E W H A L E I
U A P L A E S H S S O
E C R A B G I J T A K
S G B O U F M N B I Z
R I L O B S T E R V T
O A O C T O P U S V U
H X V N I H P L O D N
A J E L L Y F I S H A
E Z I E L T R U T K W
S G Y Y H C P T R M W
```

SEAL DOLPHIN WHALE STARFISH
LOBSTER CRAB OCTOPUS JELLYFISH
SHARK TURTLE TUNA SEAHORSE

PAGE 93

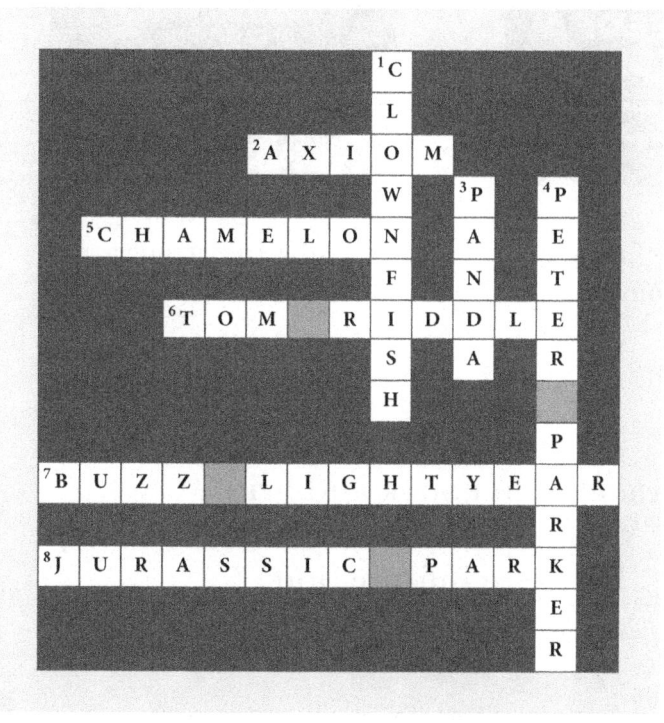

1 Down: CLWFSH
2 Across: AXIOM
3 Down: PANAHA
4 Down: PETERPARKER
5 Across: CHAMELON
6 Across: TOM RIDDLE
7 Across: BUZZ LIGHTYEAR
8 Across: JURASSIC PARK

Other Books by the Author

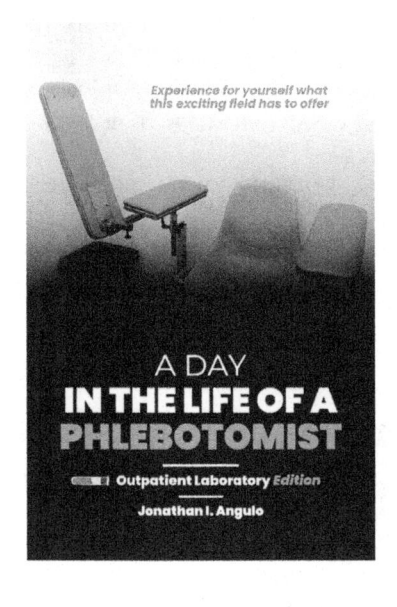

A Day in the Life of a Phlebotomist

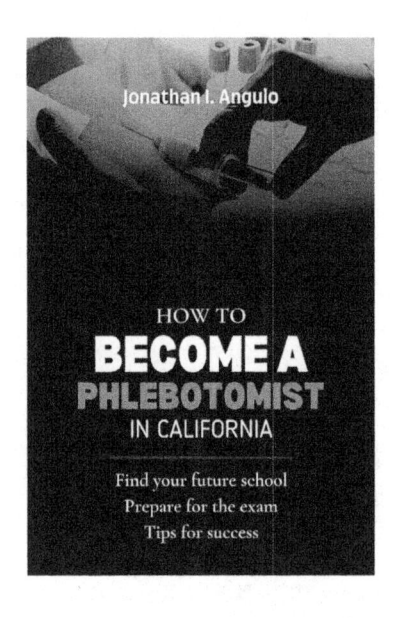

How To Become a Phlebotomist in California

Available in ebook and print.
Visit anguloauthor.com
for more information.

About the Author

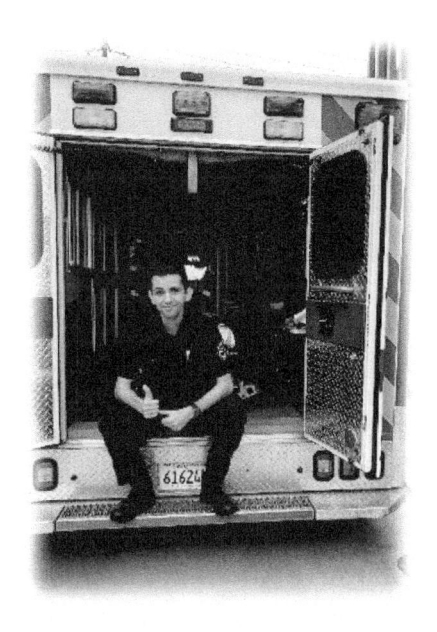

Jonathan I. Angulo began his fight against Hodgkin's Lymphoma in 2022; after months of fighting his resistant disease, he finally underwent an autologous stem cell transplant in 2023. He decided to use his own experience as a patient to create this book, hoping it would help others during their time in the hospital. Jonathan has devoted his life to helping people in need and currently volunteers at a free clinic for low-income people at his local church by serving as a board member. When he is not at work, Jonathan enjoys walking, reading, and practicing archery. He eagerly hopes to defeat his disease soon so he can go back to caring for patients and continue his education in pursuit of becoming a nurse practitioner.